NAVIGATING THE DIGITAL MAZE

Social Media, Mental Health, and Safety

NAVIGATING THE DIGITAL MAZE

Social Media, Mental Health, and Safety

HUBERT A. JEROME

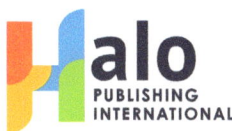

Halo
PUBLISHING
INTERNATIONAL

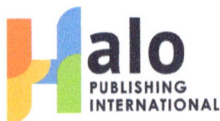

Halo Publishing International
7550 W IH-10 #800, PMB 2069,
San Antonio, TX 78229

First Edition, June 2025
ISBN: 978-1-63765-736-2
Library of Congress Control Number: 2024927542

Halo Publishing International is a self-publishing company that publishes adult fiction and non-fiction, children's literature, self-help, spiritual, and faith-based books. Do you have a book idea you would like us to consider publishing? Please visit www.halopublishing.com for more information.

To my wife, Priya, for all the love and support.

*To my daughters, Sarah and Adriana, your courage
and grit led to this book from your trials.*

*And to all the incredible people who have made me
the person I am today. You have been my strength,
my cheerleader, and my coach.*

CONTENTS

CHAPTER III
UNDERSTANDING YOUR ONLINE PERSONA   51

CHAPTER IV
THE MENTAL HEALTH CONNECTION 59

CHAPTER V
NAVIGATING CYBERBULLYING AND ONLINE HARASSMENT

CHAPTER VI
DIGITAL SAFETY 101   101

CHAPTER VII
MINDFUL SOCIAL MEDIA USE   **111**

CHAPTER VIII
COMMUNITY ENGAGEMENT IN SOCIAL
MEDIA SAFETY AND WELLNESS FOR TEENS   **119**

CHAPTER IX
BUILDING RESILIENCE
AND SELF-CARE PRACTICES

CHAPTER X
FINDING AND BUILDING
SUPPORT NETWORKS

143

LET'S CONNECT 187

CHAPTER I
THE DIGITAL AGE AND YOU

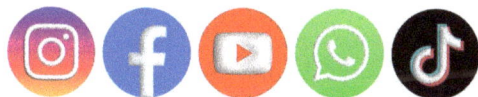

We're living in a society where we're all on our phones and screens. The importance of real human interaction is only going up.

—Mark Zuckerberg, Cofounder of Facebook

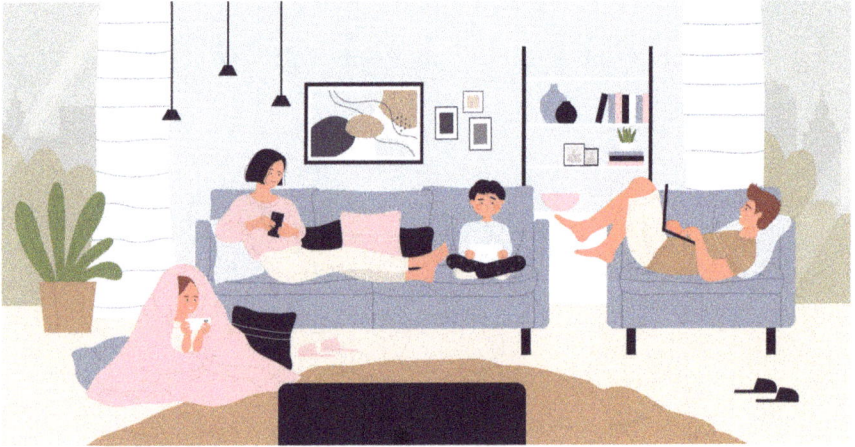

Consider a family chatting in their living room today. The soft glow of screens has replaced all conversation, board games, and shared television shows. The kids sit on the couch, each immersed in a device—one scrolls social media on a tablet, another plays an online game on a laptop, and the parents email or work on their smartphones in between glances at the latest streaming series on the big flat-screen. The tap-tap of fingers on keys and ping of message notifications fill the room, a new song of the screen.

Now, think of a family sitting together in the same place as that one from my childhood, but let's say the parents were teens then, too. The kids are probably watching the same show. The family might be listening to the radio, as I sometimes did as a child. Or maybe they are watching the television, because there is only one, and everyone in the family watches that one. Perhaps some of the kids are sprawled on the den's floor, flipping through magazines or reading a novel they checked out of the local library.

Conversations were so much freer in those days, even if punctuated by long pregnant pauses. Everyone was much more present with each other, unlike today when our lives are much more present in the digital world amongst frequently faceless digital avatars halfway around the globe.

The living rooms of pre-digital times have been replaced by the home screen of the app that has our attention for that moment. Human relationships have been transformed by the divide, and the bridge technology represents for everyone, big or small.

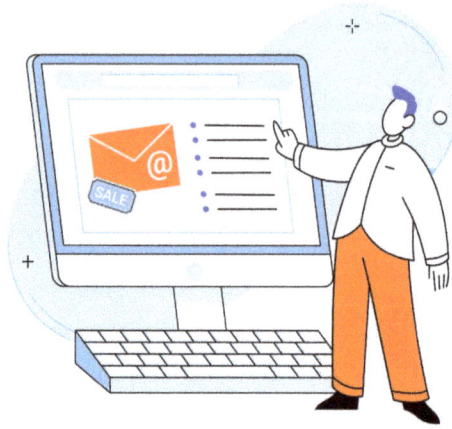

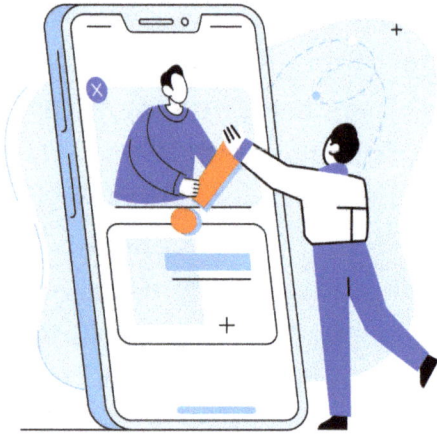

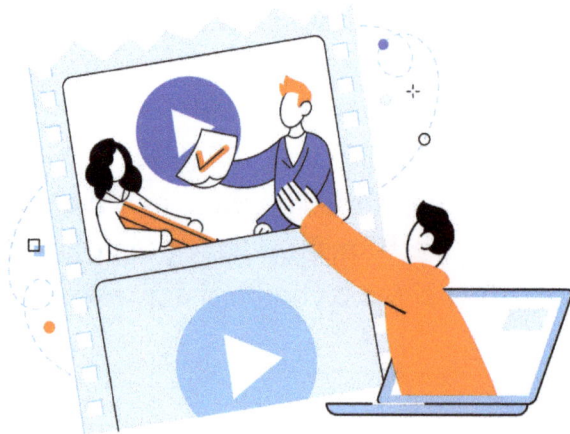

THE DIGITAL AGE

In its simplest form, the information age (or digital age) was the transition from words written on paper to letters entered via a device and viewed on an electronic screen. It began at the end of the twentieth century and continues to evolve. The development of personal computers, the internet, and mobile devices has altered how we seek, collaborate, work, learn, and consume information.

Global connectivity, the characteristic hallmark of the digital age, has empowered people and communities, joining billions of people on a worldwide scale and eliminating geographical silos. The internet, social media, instant messaging, and video conferencing services enabled a dynamic community —without geographical, cultural, or language barriers— through which information is shared in real time. And instead of users visiting libraries housed in large buildings, anyone with an internet connection can have the libraries brought to them digitally. Courses, libraries, and learning environments on the internet revolutionized education, making it accessible from everywhere so that anyone can learn new skills and acquire knowledge.

The digital age has also changed business models, resulting in e-commerce, digital payments, and the gig economy. Technologies such as wearables and mobile apps provide for health and personal monitoring. With businesses such as Amazon and Alibaba, our shopping, working, and business lives are radically changed with an emphasis on convenience and speed. Artificial intelligence and automation led this epoch, spurring progress across fields such as health care, finance, manufacturing, and more. These tools automate tasks, crunch enormous amounts of data (big data), and more, delivering previously unthinkable insight and revolutionizing business and the workforce.

Among all the digital advances and innovations, however, it has been social media networks that have changed the nature of individual interactions, information sharing, and consumption for all classes of human beings. They have opened up new spaces for speech, collective action, and social movements, but also introduced the pitfalls of disinformation (fake news), cybersecurity threats, data security issues, and mental health declines. Information overload can be caused by constant interconnectedness, internet addiction, and the age of instant gratification, particularly in young people.

The internet has also changed our basic societal fabric. The accepted norms of looking someone in the eye and shaking their hand to gauge genuineness and trust are replaced by the anonymity the digital world provides with its inherent lack of personal connections. These new social constructs (social media networks) are a leading cause of anxiety, depression, assignment of guilt, and feelings of inadequacy through constant emulation and digital overreach. Screen time affects attention span, sleep, and health more generally, but the consequences for young adults, in particular, are of growing interest.

If societies want to survive the digital era, individuals and nations must learn to embrace technologies while managing risks. As children, we were taught how to interact with other children and the etiquette of the schoolyard or local park. The vast digital playground has replaced the schoolyards and local parks, yet our children are not taught the rules or etiquette, or warned about the dangers lurking in the shadows. Online safety, literacy, and technology management are essential. If we can use technology cautiously and effectively, we can mitigate the adverse effects of technology and make the digital age work to our advantage. It is an ever-changing age whose risks and rewards demand consideration. Maintaining a well-balanced digital lifestyle assures us we're in charge of our digital life.

THE METEORIC RISE OF SOCIAL MEDIA

Social media actually got started in the 1990s with apps such as Six Degrees (1997), in which you set up your own profile and friend network. This became the origin of modern social media. During the same period, bloggers were gaining fame as well, offering a space for people to express their opinions on the internet.

Social networks such as Friendster (2002), MySpace (2003), and LinkedIn (2003), which introduced detailed profiles, media sharing, and social networking to the world in the early 2000s, refashioned how we socialize. In 2004, Facebook started as a college-only platform and quickly expanded to become the prevailing social network.

During the years 2006 to 2010, visual and microblogging networks took off. Twitter (2006) allowed microblogging—instant, short updates—and YouTube (2005) transformed the way we share and view videos. Social media entered everyday people's life.

From 2010 to 2015, mobile and visual content started taking shape with the advent of Instagram (2010) and Snapchat (2011). These sites took advantage of the smartphone revolution by placing a high value on images and videos. Social media became mobile, and more and more apps were developed for mobile use. In the world today, social media has been an established part of our culture since 2015. Sites such as TikTok (which was expanded internationally in 2018) revolutionized short video content. In 2020, Meta—the owner of Instagram—launched Instagram Reels, and YouTube launched YouTube Shorts to try to trump TikTok.

The Shares of teens who say they are online 'almost consistently' has doubled since 2014-2015

% of US teens ages 13 to 17 who say they use the internet ...

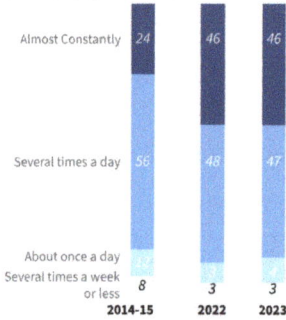

	2014-15	2022	2023
Almost Constantly	24	46	46
Several times a day	56	48	47
About once a day / Several times a week or less	8	3	3

Note: Figures may not add up to NET value.

Source: Survey of US teens conducted Sept. - Oct. 2023

"Teens, Social Media and Technology 2023"

PEW RESEARCH CENTER

Social media has become a mainstream platform for news, entertainment, and engagement and has shaped global culture, politics, and human experience. And it's always growing fast with the addition of AR filters and live streaming, along with algorithm-based content to personalize your experience. The advent of social media signifies technological development, a shift in behavior, and a continuing need for connectivity and self-expression. And it has become part of modern society—particularly for adolescents—in almost every aspect of daily life.

Teenagers have become so active with social media that some would even say it's *almost constant.* Smartphones and the internet changed the way teenagers connect and create content online. This digital culture extends to teens in the form of self-understanding, relationships, and ways of living.

GLOBAL DIGITAL OVERVIEW (2024)

	INTERNET USAGE AS % OF TOPOULTION	UNIQNE MOBILE DATA SUBRIDERVERS	SOCIAL MEDIA USER IDENTITIES
5.45 BILLION	67.1% YoY +2.3%	4.80 BILLION	5.17 BILLION

INTERNET ACCESS VIA MOBILE PHONES	INTERNET ACCESS VIA DESKTOPS	AVERAGE DAILY TIME SPENT ON INTERNET	INTERNET TRAFFIC BY MOBILE PHONES
95.9%	62,2%	6H 31M	60.71% YoY +1,9%

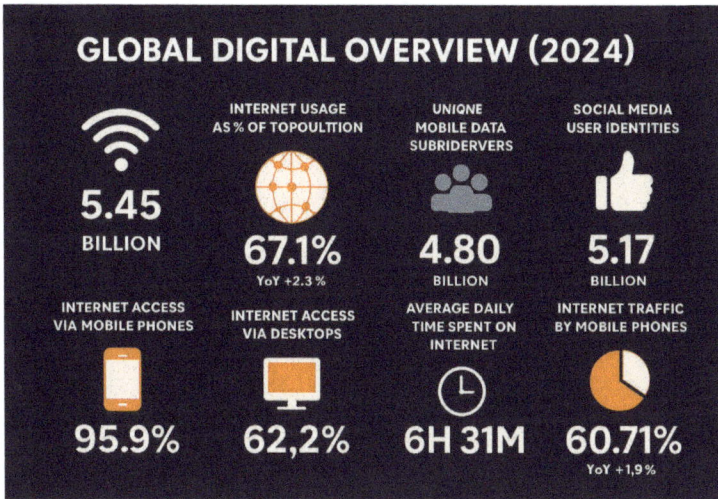

HOW DIGITAL CULTURE SHAPES MODERN TEENAGE LIFE

Adolescents use the digital world to individuate themselves on the web. Teenagers are often seen creating online avatars based on their interests and values so they can explore letting out some steam online.

Trends and romanticized representations on social media also shape adolescents' ideas of beauty, success, and social status. Such influence frequently sets high standards and pressures adolescents to achieve them.

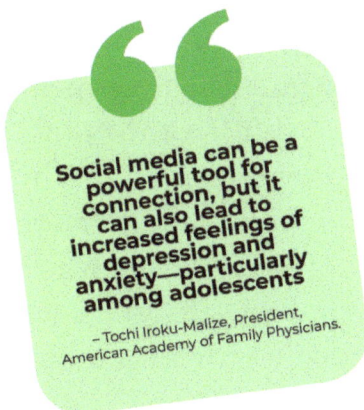

> "Social media can be a powerful tool for connection, but it can also lead to increased feelings of depression and anxiety—particularly among adolescents
>
> — Tochi Iroku-Malize, President, American Academy of Family Physicians.

Perpetual viewing of idealized lives on social media can seriously undermine adolescents' mental health. This can make them feel unworthy, more anxious, and even depressed as they pit their lives against the life they see online, feeling pressured to gain social approval.

> Teenagers have not known a world without Social Media. This is where they do thier home work, but also meeting and connecting with friends.
>
> — Dr. Sanjay Gupta, CNN 2023

Teens are on social media to get news, be educated, and have fun, as well as to organize and spread social awareness. That exposes them to other views, but also makes them vulnerable to fake news and perhaps prejudiced information.

Adolescents are profoundly affected by online marketing and millennial influencers who affect their tastes, purchases, and purchasing behavior. Digital media encourages teens to exercise their imagination and acquire skills, which allows them to participate in creative projects according to their interests and talents.

Keeping track of these effects is crucial for guiding teens toward healthier online habits and positive digital interactions. The web has revolutionized communication and attachment for teenagers and changed the social phenomenology of adolescents.

> While social media can connect teens to supportive communities, it can also expose them to bullying, harassment, and harmful content that adversely impacts their mental health.
>
> — Pew Research Center, 2022.

FREQUENCY OF USE

Nearly all teens in the US have access to a smartphone

% of US teens ages 13 to 17 who have access to the following devices at home

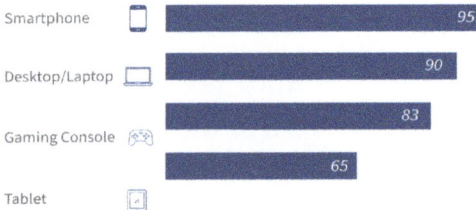

Device	%
Smartphone	95
Desktop/Laptop	90
Gaming Console	83
Tablet	65

Note: Figures may not add up to NET value.

Source: Survey of US teens conducted Sept. - Oct. 2023

"Teens, Social Media and Technology 2023"

PEW RESEARCH CENTER

Teenagers' use of social media has undergone a significant transformation with the widespread adoption of smartphones, which are now almost universally accessible to this demographic.

AVERAGE DAILY USAGE

The Shares of teens who say they are online 'almost consistently' has doubled since 2014-2015

% of US teens ages 13 to 17 who say they use the internet ...

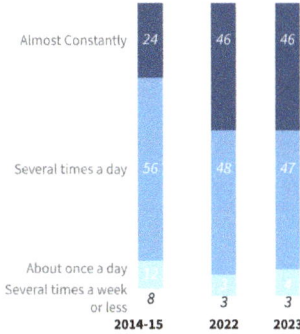

	2014-15	2022	2023
Almost Constantly	24	46	46
Several times a day	56	48	47
About once a day / Several times a week or less	8	3	3

Note: Figures may not add up to NET value.

Source: Survey of US teens conducted Sept. - Oct. 2023

"Teens, Social Media and Technology 2023"

PEW RESEARCH CENTER

There has been a huge change in the social-media use habits of adolescents now that teens are also increasingly using mobile devices. Teens spend an average of three to four hours per day on social media, and according to some studies, that can increase to seven to nine hours when combined with other online activities such as watching videos.

PLATFORM POPULARITY

Facebook, Instagram, and Snapchat are the top social media sites that teens use most often, followed by YouTube and TikTok.

Social media is used most often by teenagers—more than 80 percent—to reach out to their friends, highlighting the importance of the platform.

A majority of teens visit YouTube, TikTok daily

% of US teens ages 13 to 17 who say they visit the following sites .....

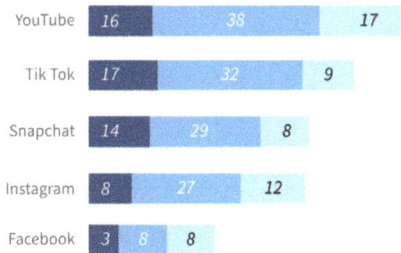

YouTube	16	38	17
Tik Tok	17	32	9
Snapchat	14	29	8
Instagram	8	27	12
Facebook	3	8	8

Note: Figures may not add up to NET value.

Source: Survey of US teens conducted Sept. - Oct. 2023

"Teens, Social Media and Technology 2023"

PEW RESEARCH CENTER

SOCIAL MEDIA AND MENTAL HEALTH

A study suggests that roughly a third of all teens believe that social media mainly affects people in their age bracket. Bullying, unrealistic expectations, peer pressure, and other effects are mentioned as especially alarming aspects of social media use.

More than 70 percent of all adolescents also claim that their screens interfere with their sleep. It is also true that if teens use social media over three hours per day, they are more likely to show symptoms of depression and anxiety. Asked if they could drop social media, 54 percent of all teens say that this would be a challenge.

54% of teens say it would be hard to give up social media

% of US teens who say the amount of time they spend on social media is .....

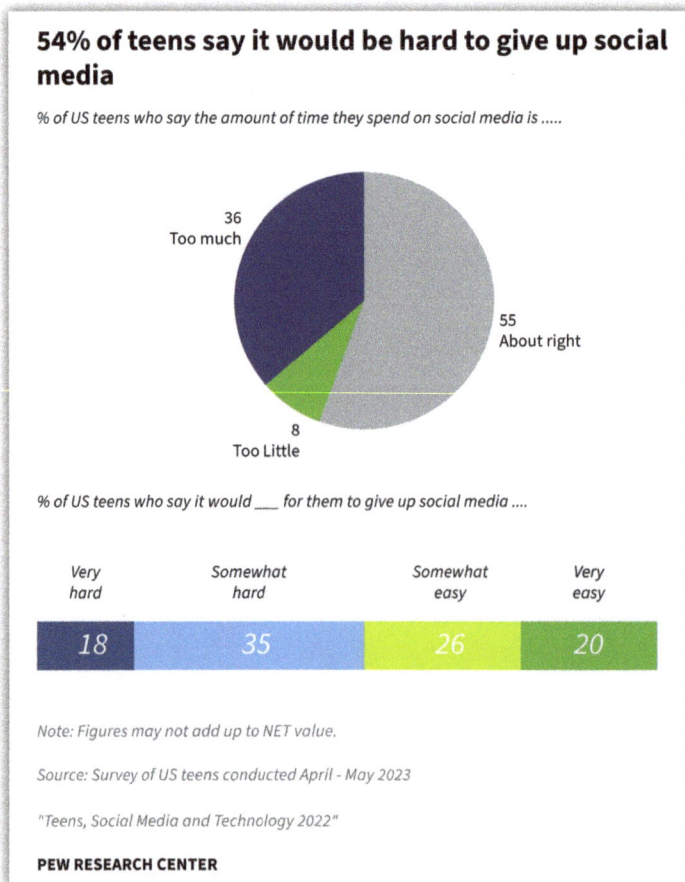

36
Too much

55
About right

8
Too Little

% of US teens who say it would ___ for them to give up social media ....

Very hard	Somewhat hard	Somewhat easy	Very easy
18	35	26	20

Note: Figures may not add up to NET value.

Source: Survey of US teens conducted April - May 2023

"Teens, Social Media and Technology 2022"

PEW RESEARCH CENTER

CHAPTER II

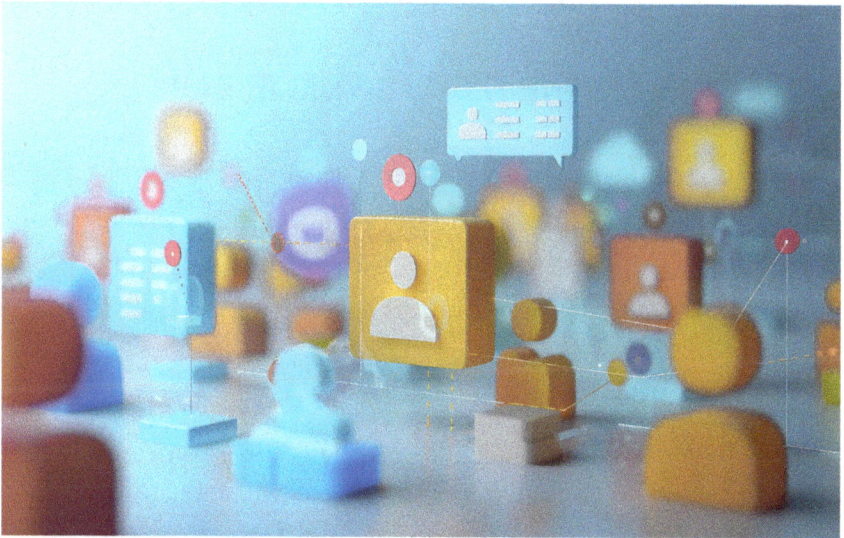

The challenge for social media platforms today
is balancing innovation with responsibility, ensuring
that technology enhances human connection
rather than undermines it.

—Sundar Pichai, CEO of Google

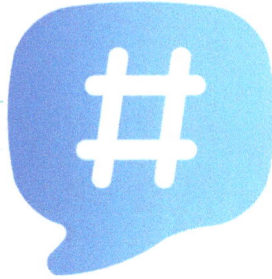

WELCOME TO THE DIGITAL THEME PARK

It's a virtual amusement park with ever-changing rides. There's TikTok, a roller-coaster ride through fifteen-second dancing fads, and then there is Facebook, the giant Ferris wheel that seems to be slowing down to almost a standstill these days, but great for family updates and that picture of your kids in first grade.

And this digital theme park is ever-changing. The list of attractions is a long one: Facebook, TikTok, Instagram, Twitter (now known as X for, you know, the edgy rebrand), LinkedIn, Snapchat, Threads. And on it goes.

Every site contains its own vibe. Instagram is all about the filtered snapshot of what life looks like when you control everything…and a cup of coffee looks like the *Mona Lisa*.

TikTok feels as if it is a nonstop talent show in which everyone is either dancing, singing, lip-synching, or being funny in a way that lasts all of five seconds.

Snapchat was/is fleeting and friendly about sharing an inside joke that dissipates after five seconds. LinkedIn is people donning their sackcloths and cardboard cutouts of ties at their desks, sharing career milestones and inspirational quotes. And Twitter (X) feels as if it is that one noise-making party guest ranting about something you don't care about, throwing out a quip to get everyone laughing, or tossing a little bit of dynamite on a can of gasoline.

Social media is a beach where the tide never stops moving. It's about what's new or the next big thing. It is about #BeReal this week and then next week trying to discern if Threads will work out or not. You begin to think you've got your finger on what's hot, only to have the sand slip out from beneath your feet and a wave of new trending content or features pull you in a completely new direction.

While there is some good in social media, with the good comes the bad. For every virtual panacea, there is its nemesis; the social media amusement park has a haunted house, after all. Misinformation lurks in dark corners…and sometimes hides in plain sight, waiting for the right moment to pounce, sometimes triggering real-world catastrophe. Privacy breaches are possessed scarecrows that haunt the woods, luring you to reveal more than you intended.

Cyberbullying is that one party guest who never feels welcome and persists in making everyone else feel equally unwelcome. Being on twenty-four seven—to post, to stay sexy, or to seem happier than everyone else's brilliant, uneventful lives—can take its toll on the psyche, potentially driving people further apart than together.

But even through all of the stutters, hiccups, haunted-house flashes, and uh-ohs, the bottom line is that nobody really wants to take social media down. Nobody really wants to let go of their connection to the world.

This is where revolutions start, after all, where memes are born, where someone's cat becomes more famous than most media actors. It is how people connect across continents, how people share their art and their voices and their lives, all through a series of beeps and taps and flashes on a screen. Businesses are booming, creative talent finds its following, and everyone—celebrities, attention solicitors, and that videographer in your neighborhood—is a proprietor of his or her own stage, and anything and everything that flows from that creative portal might be necessary for their pitch-perfect soundtrack.

Being able to navigate such a landscape is sometimes slippery and potentially hazardous if the steering is careless and ill-intentioned, but you just might catch a butterfly if you're quick enough, thoughtful, and responsible. Ultimately, we would all do well to remember that we are as much a part of the landscape as the medium that surrounds us. It is one of those out-of-body experiences in which you look back on your lives. It might be best to take a moment every now and then to hop off the roller coaster and climb into the Ferris wheel car, or maybe stop and enjoy the fried Snickers bars along with the view!

The social media landscape is a constantly evolving digital environment that encompasses various platforms, tools, and communities designed for communication, content sharing, and social interaction. Major platforms like Facebook, Instagram, TikTok, Twitter (X), LinkedIn, and Snapchat dominate this space, each catering to different audiences and purposes—from personal networking and entertainment to professional connections and brand marketing.

This landscape is characterized by rapid innovation and changing user dynamics, with new features, trends, and platforms emerging regularly. It has transformed how individuals and businesses interact, offering unprecedented opportunities for connection, self-expression, and real-time engagement on a global scale. However, the social media landscape also presents challenges, such as the spread of misinformation, privacy concerns, cyberbullying, and an adverse impact on mental health.

As platforms continuously adapt to user demands and technological advances, the social media landscape remains a powerful force that shapes public discourse, consumer behavior, and cultural trends. Therefore, it is essential for users to navigate this space mindfully and responsibly.

YOUTUBE

Launched in 2005, You-Tube is a video-sharing platform where users can upload, watch, and interact with videos across various genres, including vlogs, tutorials, music, gaming, education, and more. It is the world's second most visited website, just after Google.

YouTube Key Features

Channels and Subscriptions
Users can create channels to share content, build audiences, and subscribe to others for updates.

Monetization
Creators can earn revenue through ads, channel memberships, and merchandise sales.

Live Streaming:
Allows creators to engage with their audience in real-time.

YouTube Shorts
Competes with TikTok, offering short-form, vertical videos.

YouTube Algorithm and Content-Prioritization Factors

YouTube uses a recommendation algorithm that combines machine learning, user-behavior analysis, and content meta-data, using the following **content-prioritization factors:**

Watch Time: YouTube prioritizes videos that keep viewers watching for more extended periods, as its goal is to keep users on the platform.

Engagement Metrics: Likes, comments, shares, and click-through rates influence how videos are recommended.

Personalization: YouTube customizes the home page and suggests videos based on users' watch history, search queries, and previously engaged content.

Recency and Relevance: New and relevant videos are slightly boosted, particularly if they concern trending topics.

Effect on Teens: The algorithm often pushes similar content, potentially leading teens into echo chambers of repetitive or extreme content.

Adjusting Your Feed

The ways in which you can customize your YouTube feed are:

Watch and Engage with Preferred Content: The algorithm learns from what you watch and engage with, so focus on videos that align with your interests.

YouTube Impact on teens

EDUCATION RESOURCE
To learn, from DIY projects to academic help

INFLUENCER CULTURE
Follow influencers and creators who shape trends, opinions, and consumer habits

MENTAL HEALTH
Positive content can be inspiring, but unrealistic portrayals of life can lead to social comparison.

Use "Not Interested" or "Don't Recommend Channel" Options: When you see videos or channels you don't like, click on these options to teach YouTube what you prefer.

Manage Subscriptions: Subscribe to channels that consistently provide value, and manage notifications to see new content from your favorite creators.

User Demographics

YouTube is a widely popular platform utilized by people across all age groups. Notably, many teenagers consistently engage with the platform's content. Recent statistics indicate that approximately 77 percent of individuals aged fifteen to twenty-five are active users of YouTube.

INSTAGRAM

Instagram, launched in 2010 and acquired by Facebook (now Meta) in 2012, is a photo- and video-sharing platform focused on visual storytelling, self-expression, and social interaction.

Instagram Key Feature

Posts and Stories
Shared images, videos, and ephemeral stories that disappear after 24 hours.

Reels
Short, engaging videos similar to TikTok's format, designed for discoverability.

Direct Messages (DMs)
Private communication between users.

Online Store
Purchases made directly from posts.

Instagram Algorithm and Content-Prioritization Factors

Instagram's algorithm uses machine learning and data analysis to personalize the feed and stories, and to explore pages and reels. The content-prioritization factors they use are:

Engagement Signals: Posts that users have previously liked, commented on, saved, or shared are more likely to appear at the top of their feed.

Relationships: Instagram prioritizes content from accounts with which users frequently interact, such as friends, family, and favorite influencers.

Relevancy and Interests: Instagram tracks what users engage with most (for example, fashion, fitness, memes) and pushes similar content to their feed and explore page.

Timeliness: More recent posts are given a slight edge, but not at the expense of personalized relevance.

User Activity: What users see is influenced by how long users spend on Instagram and the type of content they engage with.

Effect on Teens: This prioritization can reinforce body-image issues, peer pressure, and the pursuit of likes, often leading to a cycle of comparison and validation-seeking behavior.

Adjusting Your Feed

The ways in which you can customize your Instagram feed are:

Interact with Desired Content: Like, save, and comment on posts that resonate with you. Instagram uses these signals to prioritize content in your feed.

Mute or Unfollow Accounts: If an account's content is no longer relevant, you can mute it (to hide posts and stories without actually unfollowing the account) or unfollow it to stop seeing their content altogether.

Explore Page Customization: On the Explore page, long press on posts you don't like and select Not Interested to adjust the types of posts shown to you.

User Demographics

This platform is hugely popular among the younger demographic, with 71 percent of all teenagers frequenting it.

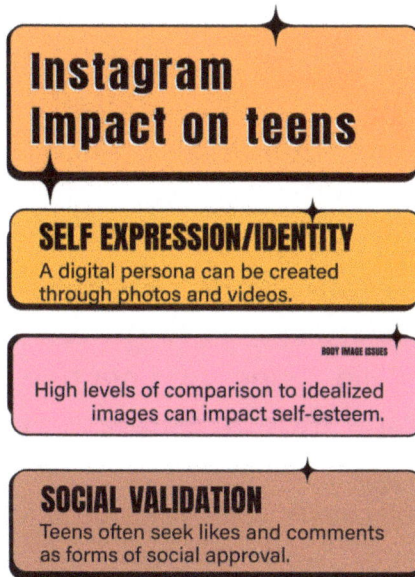

Instagram Impact on teens

SELF EXPRESSION/IDENTITY
A digital persona can be created through photos and videos.

BODY IMAGE ISSUES
High levels of comparison to idealized images can impact self-esteem.

SOCIAL VALIDATION
Teens often seek likes and comments as forms of social approval.

In 2019, a low-key social media assault began on Instagram that would sweep the world in the following months. There was just one simple photograph of...well, an egg. The image was posted to an account with the handle @world_record_egg, accompanied by the summation "Let's set a world record together and get the most-liked post on Instagram. Beating the current world record holders, Kylie Jenner (18 million)!" Bug-eyed and cozily white, the egg itself meanly stared back at us. When the post went up, few of us would have bet that the egg would take the world by storm. After all, the previous world record for the most-liked image on Instagram was 18 million likes, set in February 2018 by Kylie Jenner and her newborn daughter. Hard to imagine that an egg was ever supposed to beat this.

The Instagram community nonetheless rallied behind the @worldrecordegg post, and in the space of just a few weeks, the account's humble picture broke the world record for the most-liked Instagram post, garnering more than 55 million likes in a matter of weeks. The 2019 egg explosion was an internet oddity. For a few brief sun-dappled weeks, everyone seemed to be egg crazy in 2019. The simplicity of sneaky-egg domination was nevertheless a bracing wake-up call for those of us who had become trapped in the digital world. Anything can go viral in the electronic vacuum of the internet.

TIKTOK

TikTok, launched internationally in 2018 by ByteDance, is a short-form video platform that has rapidly gained popularity, especially among younger users, due to its highly engaging and personalized content.

TikTok Algorithm and Content-Prioritization Factors

TikTok's algorithm is highly advanced. It uses artificial intelligence (AI) and deep-learning models to create the highly personalized For You Page (FYP) using the following content-prioritization factors:

User Interactions: Likes, shares, comments, follows, and watch duration play significant roles in what videos are pushed to a user's FYP.

Video Information: Hashtags, captions, sounds, and content types are analyzed to match videos with user preferences.

Device and Account Settings: Location, language, device type, and account settings help tailor the FYP experience.

Watch Behavior: The algorithm closely monitors watch time. Videos watched until the end or replayed are heavily favored.

Content Freshness: New content from lesser-known creators can be boosted to test its engagement potential with new audiences.

Effect on Teens: The hyperpersonalized FYP can lead to rapid exposure to trends, sometimes promoting harmful content or unrealistic lifestyle portrayals that can affect mental health.

Adjusting your Feed

The ways in which you can customize your TikTok feed are:

Engage with Positive Content: Like and comment on videos you enjoy. TikTok's algorithm heavily relies on engagement metrics to curate your For You Page (FYP).

TikTok Impact on teens

CREATIVITY & SELF EXPRESSION
Creative content creation and participation in global trends are encouragd.

VIRAL INFLUENCE
High levels of comparison to idealized images can impact self-esteem.

MENTAL HEALTH
The fast pace and pressure to go viral can be overwhelming.

Hold Down on Videos and Select "Not Interested": This feature lets TikTok know what kind of videos you'd rather not see, refining your FYP recommendations.

Follow Hashtags and Creators: Following hashtags that match your interests and creators whose content you consistently enjoy will enhance the relevance of your feed.

User Demographics

TikTok has gained immense popularity among teenagers, with 58 percent of its user base belonging to this demographic. The platform's youthful and energetic atmosphere has successfully captivated millions of teenagers worldwide.

SNAPCHAT

Launched in 2011, Snapchat is a multimedia messaging app known for its disappearing content, private messaging, and augmented reality (AR) features, like filters and lenses.

Snapchat Key Features

Snaps and Stories
Short-lived photos and videos that disappear after viewing or after 24 hours.

Snap Map
Shows friends' locations and highlights popular places.

Streaks
Tracks the number of consecutive days users have exchanged messages, encouraging daily interaction.

AR Lenses
Interactive lenses and filters that add fun effects to selfies and videos.

Snapchat Algorithm and Content-Prioritization Factors

Snapchat uses algorithms to prioritize content in the Discover feed, Stories, and personalized Snap Maps, mainly based on user interaction and engagement. The content prioritization factors used to do this are:

Engagement: Similar to other platforms, engagement metrics (taps, views, shares) determine the prominence of Snaps and Stories.

Friend Interactions: The Snap Map and Stories prioritize content from friends whom users frequently interact with, emphasizing close social connections.

Location-Based Content: Local and regional trends are factored into what appears on Discover and Maps, making it location sensitive.

Media Partnerships: Content from verified accounts, celebrities, and media partners is often given greater visibility.

Effect on Teens: The emphasis on close connections can amplify social dynamics such as peer pressure, fear of missing out (FOMO), and the drive to maintain "streaks" for validation.

Adjusting your Feed

The ways in which you can customize your feed are:

Adjust Discover Content: Tap and hold on Discover content you don't like and select See Less Like This to adjust future recommendations.

Manage Subscriptions: Subscribe to creators and channels you find entertaining or informative. Avoid irrelevant content.

Snapchat Impact on teens

PRIVACY AND EPHEMERALITY
Temporary nature appeals to teens offers a sense of privacy.

SOCIAL INTERACTION
High levels of comparison to idealized images can impact self-esteem.

PEER PRESSURE AND FOMO
Streaks can create pressure to maintain constant contact, leading to FOMO.

Customize Snap Map Settings: You can adjust what content you see based on location by controlling whom you interact with on Snap Map and managing visibility settings.

User Demographics

Snapchat is a popular social media platform, especially among the younger demographic. Statistical data indicates that 75 percent of its users are aged thirteen to thirty-four, solidifying its position as the leading platform for teenagers and young adults.

IMPACT ACROSS PLATFORMS

Social Validation: In the contemporary digital landscape, it is increasingly common for teenagers to yearn for validation and affirmation. The most common method for gauging their worth is by quantifying their likes, views, and followers on various social media platforms. This persistent pursuit of online approval often plays a substantial role in shaping their self-esteem and overall sense of self-worth, potentially contributing to both positive and negative outcomes.

Exposure to Diverse Content: Platforms are important in sharing many sources of information and forming communities, which are extremely helpful to teens. But it's important to understand that those same sites are also a great way to mislead and poison teens. Without proper controls, these algorithms can result in sending children to inappropriate, radical, or harmful material. Therefore, we need to ensure digital literacy and mindful engagement are top priorities for adolescents to be safe online and interact in a responsible manner.

Echo Chambers and Filter Bubbles: Algorithms affect how we engage with the internet by capping our experiences and habits. Yet these algorithms can create even more societal biases by keeping us out of other people's perspectives and creating echo chambers in which reality gets distorted. This has an open-ended effect, from how we read the news to how we socialize.

Mental Health Challenges: The fact that people check social media without supervision or constraints can cause anxiety, depression, and loneliness. Therefore, social media usage must be approached with deliberate intent and consideration of its consequences on mental health. It means paying attention to what you are reading and watching and the effects on your mood and mental state. By using social media responsibly, people can minimize the risk to their mental well-being and create a better, more positive relationship with social media. These platforms each play unique roles in teens' lives, shaping their social interactions, self-expression, and world and self-perceptions.

GENERAL TIPS FOR ALL PLATFORMS

Adjusting your social media feeds in the following ways can improve your experience and promote mental well-being by reducing exposure to irrelevant or harmful content:

Engage Mindfully: The more you engage with content (likes, comments, shares), the more the algorithm will prioritize similar posts. Engage with the content you genuinely enjoy or find valuable. Avoid interacting with hostile or irrelevant posts.

Unfollow or Mute Accounts: If you find certain accounts no longer align with your interests or negatively affect you, unfollow or mute them. This will help declutter your feed and reduce exposure to unwanted content.

Use See Less or Not Interested Options: Most platforms can hide specific content types or sources. Use these features to indicate what you don't want to see, guiding the algorithm to adjust accordingly.

Adjust Notifications: Customize your notification settings to only alert you about essential interactions. This will reduce distractions and help you stay focused on what matters.

Curate Your Follow Lists: Regularly review and update whom you follow. Focus on accounts that inspire, educate, or positively entertain you. Unfollow those that no longer serve your interests.

CHAPTER III
UNDERSTANDING YOUR ONLINE PERSONA

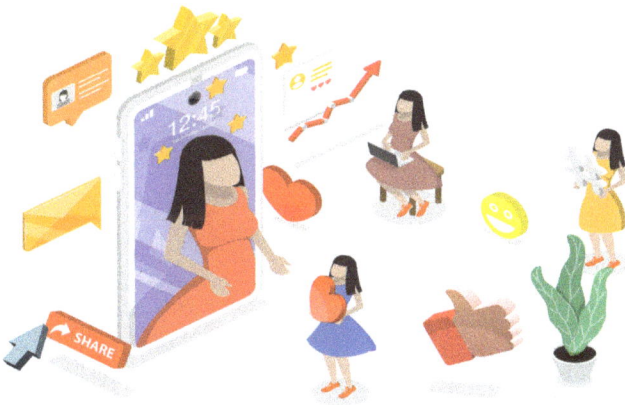

Understanding your online persona is about being aware of the digital footprint you leave behind —every post, comment, and interaction contributes to your public narrative.

—Jay Shetty, Author and Former Monk

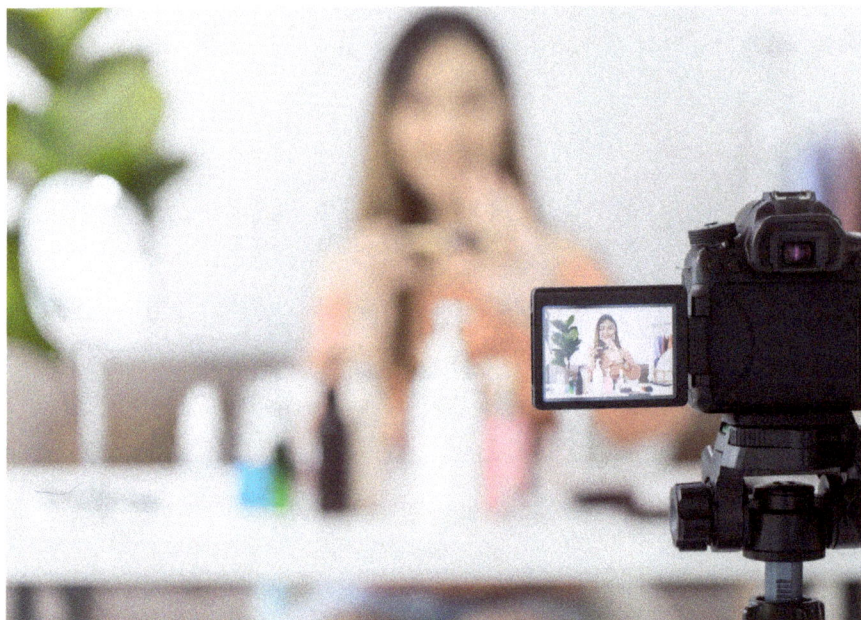

In 2006, the web was awash in chatter about a young woman, age seventeen or so, named Lonelygirl15. Each week, Bree, as she was called, posted video blogs online (called vlogs), revealing details about her life as a bizarrely cool, homeschooled teen facing all manner of angst and friend drama, the occasional family kerfuffle as well. Bree's YouTube channel grew slowly but steadily and became the most subscribed YouTube channel in June 2006. Fans were captivated by her sense of humor and honesty. And then, after three months of storytelling, news broke on the Lonelygirl15 website. Bree was fake. She was an act. An actress named Jessica Rose was actually behind the Lonelygirl15 persona, who was a carefully crafted fictional character. The so-called phenomenon grew to its most extensive viewership in 2007 until it fizzled.

In 2016, TikTok, the popular video app owned by Byte-Dance, saw the arrival of a mysterious new influencer, @LilMiquela. Her photoshop-smooth skin, pastel outfits, and "I meant what I said" captions surrounding meticulously curated lifestyle posts accumulated millions of followers—and viewers who gasped in surprise that Miquela wasn't real. She is a CGI influencer (yes, that is an actual job title) created for a company called Brud, by Trevor McFedries and Sara DeCou. Miquela follows real people, plays around with gender-fluid avant-garde ideas, promotes a unique collection of Prada sunglasses, complains about politicians, and records rap songs—while her devoted fans discuss whether her existence is real. How much of online life is real? What does it mean to follow Lil Miquela if she is not a human person? Miquela trains our focus on the mash-up of the real and the simulated, stimulating conversations about how the boundary nucleating this cultural conjunction is disappearing. Younger generations balance between a simultaneous immersion in and alienation from the digital world—it would be unthinkable, for many TikTok users, to not live half or even most of their lives online. Lil Miquela's TikTok videos weave narratives about fame, romance, power, and friendship—filling an everyday gap in narratives of selfhood. Miquela's ability to be something interesting despite being "utterly empty" or "nonexistent" begs us to ask: Does it matter if an online persona is, technically, not human?

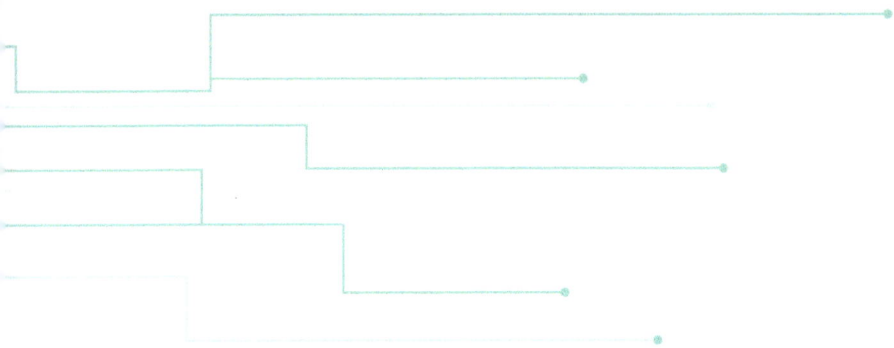

An online persona is a person's identity, personality, or character that they have created on the internet, through social media, websites, forums, and so forth. A digital identity, unlike one's offline self, can be designed and tailored to emphasize certain dimensions of personality, ideology, or way of life, while minimizing others. This digital persona can be extremely authentic representations of an individual's real self, or purely fictional fabricated avatars created for particular uses or audiences.

Creating an online character is about the person you choose to project yourself to be in your posts, comments, likes, and interactions. You can, for example, craft your digital identity to look more professional on LinkedIn, more social on Instagram, or more vocal on Twitter. This carefully cultivated presence, in turn, can influence other people and offer you opportunities, friendships, and authority. Although an online presence allows a person to voice their own creativity and engage with larger circles, it also has downsides. An inconsistent online and offline self is bound to cause conflicts or anxiety at home, particularly in the case of projecting an unrealistic avatar. Also, digital footprints are always there; therefore, old or deleted material can be rediscovered both personally and professionally.

In order to know and take control of your online presence, you need to be careful what you publish, what you interact with, and what your online activity means in the long run. If you're authentic, responsible, and aware of privacy settings, you can keep your online identity positive and steady, and it will match your values and intentions.

Creating Authentic Online Persona

- ✓ Be True to Your Values and Interests
- ✓ Avoid Overediting and Filters
- ✓ Use Your Own Voice
- ✓ Share Both Highs and Lows
- ✓ Set Boundaries on What You Share
- ✓ Engage Authentically with Others
- ✓ Post What Feels Right, Not Just What Gets Likes
- ✓ Stay Consistent Over Time

THE PRESSURE TO CURATE A PERFECT IMAGE

Adolescents frequently experience a strong urge to portray an idealized image of themselves on social media platforms. They tend to share carefully constructed content, including their proudest achievements, selectively edited photographs, and only the most positive moments from their lives.

The act of constructing one's image and persona places immense pressure to present an idealized version of oneself, resulting in heightened stress, anxiety, and fear of being judged if one falls short of these self-imposed standards.

HIGHLIGHT REEL VERSUS EVERYDAY LIFE

There's a tendency on social media to put more emphasis on vacations, celebrations, and happiness, and not on customary challenges, failures, and humdrum daily activities. This

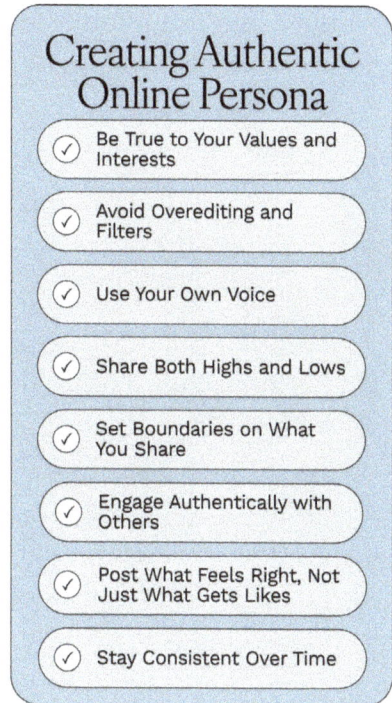

selective sharing can leave teens feeling underappreciated and instill in them a fear of missing out (FOMO).

And filters, manipulations, and unrealistic expectations in social media platforms also help to distort perceptions of the world. These enhancements make for unattainable comparisons and unreachable standards, promoting unhappiness and insecurity.

FILTERS, EDITS, AND UNREALISTIC STANDARDS

Teenagers often use filters, editing software, and other digital tools to manipulate their body image to give a vision of who they could be or wish to be, and this idealized self does not always align with reality. It's this everyday exposure to images that saturates their sense of self, making them unsatisfied with their bodies and promoting unrealistic expectations of beauty and perfection. We have to acknowledge these forces and offer the support needed to help young people establish a healthy and realistic sense of self.

SEEKING VALIDATION THROUGH LIKES AND COMMENTS

Adolescents often measure their self-worth by the number of likes, comments, or followers they receive on social media, creating a connection between online approval and their value. When their posts don't get the response they had hoped for, this can decrease their self-esteem, driving them to constantly seek validation from others.

Masking True Emotions: In contemporary culture, social media platforms frequently incentivize adolescents to curate a facade of happiness and positivity, even during periods of personal turmoil, stress, or mental health dilemmas. This compulsion to conceal genuine emotions can engender feelings of seclusion, as adolescents may perceive themselves as the sole individuals grappling with adversities, consequently diminishing their inclination to seek assistance.

Influencer Culture and Aspiration: The portrayal of lifestyles by influencers often creates an illusion of effortless glamour, excitement, and success, which could lead to the development of unrealistic aspirations among teenagers. Constant comparison with influencers may trigger feelings of inadequacy and foster materialistic desires, potentially diminishing teenagers' appreciation for their achievements and impacting their self-esteem.

Disconnection from Authentic Self: The ongoing effort to cultivate an online identity may lead adolescents to become disconnected from their genuine selves, prioritizing external perceptions over internal authenticity. Consequently, this disconnection may prompt uncertainty regarding personal identity, culminating in heightened apprehension related to acceptance and self-worth.

Ways to Encourage Authenticity and Balance

Promote Self-Awareness: It's important to help teenagers recognize that everybody has imperfections and challenges that may not be apparent on social media. Encouraging self-reflection and authenticity in their use of social media platforms can help them develop a healthier and more honest approach to online interactions.

Limit Social Media Comparisons: Remember that what people share on social media is often just a highlight reel and doesn't reflect the whole reality of their lives. It's essential to remind teenagers to appreciate and take pride in their accomplishments and experiences, no matter how big or small they may seem.

Foster Real-Life Connections: Encourage teenagers to focus on nurturing and prioritizing deep, meaningful relationships with people in real life. Spend time on activities and hobbies that make you feel good about yourself, regardless of how many likes or comments you get online.

SUMMARY AND TO-DO LIST

This mismatch between how someone presents themselves on social media and what they really are can be devastating for adolescents' mental health and self-esteem. As teenagers constantly evaluate themselves against other people's highly curated, overly idealized social media avatars, the negative self-image can cause feelings of unworthiness, anxiety, and low self-esteem. Yet with more conscious and authentic

Smart Tips

Assessing Your Digital Persona

1. REGULARLY REVIEW YOUR ONLINE PRESENCE

2. CONSIDER THE IMPACT OF YOUR WORDS!

3. UNDERSTAND PRIVACY VS. PUBLICITY

4. EVALUATE ENGAGEMENT TRENDS

5. SEEK FEEDBACK FROM TRUSTED SOURCES

social media use, teens can grow to accept themselves more and embrace who they are, which will create a healthier self-image. This can mitigate the harms of comparison and overreach, which in turn can lead to a healthier, happier online experience for teens.

CHAPTER IV

THE MENTAL HEALTH CONNECTION

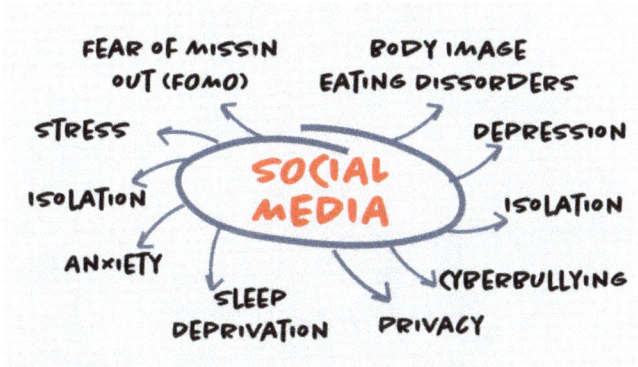

Social media has the power to connect us but also the potential to isolate us. It's crucial to set boundaries that protect our mental well-being.

—Dr. Vivek Murthy, 2022 US Surgeon General

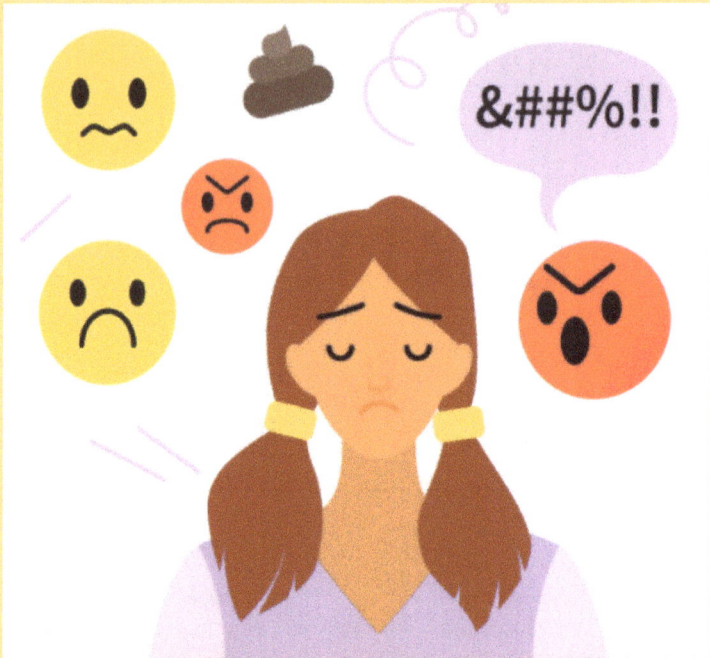

In 2017, singer and actress Selena Gomez talked about her own mental illness and social media use. One of Instagram's most-followed users at the time, Selena exposed how Instagram was hurting her. And although she had the perfect life online, she acknowledged publicly that rummaging through her feed made her anxious, lonely, and self-conscious. "It's not real," she told an interviewer and revealed that she never felt the connection between what she was posting and what she was feeling. Selena opted to take a long hiatus from social media and left it in the care of her team. Her open confession reached millions of fans and reminded the world of how egregious and taxing on the mind social media can be. She spoke to a growing fear of the modern individual—how hard the constant comparison is and how the search for digital perfection can hurt your self-confidence and mental health.

In 2021, British actress Emma Stone revealed why online production makes her life feel out of control even though she herself rarely uses social media. Stone told Vanity Fair magazine in February that she stays off Instagram or Twitter because "it's scary... Just seeing lives, even other people's lives, through a screen—I don't know; it feels a little anxiety-inducing." She said, "Even seeing other people's lives, in a way, that's enough to make me feel bad about myself or insecure about something." She admitted that on a larger scale, social media "makes other people feel like they have to look a certain way... I don't know; it's a lot, and we're already so...screwed in reality. It can throw things off, for sure." In the interview, Stone emphasized the need for boundaries: "Even a curated view into others' lives can be overwhelming for anyone suffering from anxiety." Her decision to opt out of social media is part of a growing trend of public figures leaving social media to avoid burnout and be kind to their psyches. It impressed the vulnerable millions who experience the same pressures in a world consumed by comparison.

The number of people with mental health issues is increasing 13 percent annually across the globe, according to recent studies. Both anxiety and depression are most prevalent, affecting 264 million and 280 million individuals worldwide, respectively. Mental health and social media are inherently linked, entangled, and can have both positive and negative consequences for the user, especially adolescents and young adults. And on the plus side, social media is a way to feel a sense of community, connection, and usefulness; it is a place to share, gain mental health tools, and locate support groups that aren't accessible elsewhere. These platforms can be useful for advocacy, for spreading knowledge about mental health issues, and for breaking stigmas by openly conversing.

But social media is also a serious threat to mental health. Having to constantly see polished and perfect content can make you feel bad, anxious, and depressed, and make you look at others' lives as if they had it all together. Online bullying, harassment, and insecurity needing attention and acceptance contribute to stress levels and poor self-esteem. What's more, screen time and the addictive effects of social media can make it hard to sleep, diminish face-to-face interaction, and leave us feeling lonely and alone.

Balancing social media use with healthy boundaries is crucial for protecting mental health. This includes setting time limits, curating a positive feed, engaging mindfully, and taking regular breaks to disconnect. Understanding the connection between mental health and social media empowers users to leverage its benefits while mitigating its downsides, fostering a healthier relationship with the digital world.

SOCIAL COMPARISON THEORY

Psychologist Leon Festinger formulated this theory in 1954; it argues that people judge their social and personal worth from the perspective of others. This social comparison theory helps to explain why people feel an inclination to compare themselves to others, especially in terms of skills, achievements, looks, and status. Social comparison can be positive or negative, and each perspective has different effects on self-regard and motivation.

Upward Comparison

This occurs when individuals compare themselves to someone they perceive as superior in some way, such as being more successful, attractive, talented, or better off. While upward comparisons can inspire motivation and self-improvement, they often lead to feelings of inadequacy, low self-esteem, and dissatisfaction, especially when the perceived gap in status feels unbridgeable.

Downward Comparison

By contrast, downward comparison involves comparing yourself with others who are deemed to be worse off. This can lead to a boost in self-esteem, and a sense of relief or gratitude, and a tendency to feel good about your life. But it can also breed complacency and delusional superiority.

Motivation and Self-Assessment

Social comparison is also an important aspect of self-assessment and motivation. In comparing themselves to others, people are trying to determine their place in society, and it can affect what they want to do, how they behave, and what they want to achieve. For instance, students could compare their grades with those of others to see where they stand, which can inspire them to try harder or discourage them and instill a sense of futility.

Implications for the Digital Age

Social comparison theory applies to the digital world in particular since social media offers new opportunities for comparison. Instagram, Facebook, and TikTok are the places where we are constantly posting edited versions of our lives, full of successes, beauty, and luxury. Such constant exposure to fantasy images can exacerbate upward expectations, resulting in inferiority, fear, and depression, especially in adolescents and young adults.

Coping with Social Comparison

Learning about social comparison theory can help individuals understand how these comparisons are negatively impacting their mental health. By working on self-improvement, being realistic about one's goals, and managing social media feeds to minimize the onset of catalyst posts, social comparison can have an inhibitory impact. You can also shift the attention from external praise to internal delight through mindfulness, self-compassion, and gratitude exercises.

Constant comparison can make users feel insecure and suffer from low-esteem and depression, particularly when users feel less successful, attractive, or popular than others.

REWARD SYSTEMS AND DOPAMINE RELEASE

Both reward systems and the release of dopamine are key components of pleasure, motivation, and learning in the brain. Dopamine is the feel-good chemical that floods the brain with rewarding information. This biological process reinforces behavior by creating pleasure and contentment, so we repeat over and over again the behaviors that made us feel good—eating, hanging out with friends, completing an action, etc.

Normal actions such as eating, moving, and interacting release dopamine, but our modern surroundings have opened up fresh and often greater sources of stimulation. Addictive drugs, alcohol, and nicotine take control of the reward circuit by engorging the brain with artificial dopamine, generating a riot of pleasure. Over time, the brain begins to require more and more dopamine for the same effect, creating dependency and addiction. Even behaviors such as gambling and wasting time online can create the same types of responses. The anticipation of reward is as addictive as the reward itself. Social media, games, and other online media have been engineered to take advantage of this reward system by delivering fast, repeated doses of dopamine. Every like, comment, and notification elicits some small dopamine release, which engages users and frequently leads to addiction.

Learning more about dopamine and reward systems can guide actions that are so heavily based on the availability of immediate satisfaction. Mindfulness, long-term intentions, and concentrating on things that reward in deeper, more rewarding ways can offset dopamine production. Exercise, healthy sleep, and limited digital-screen time are convenient ways to balance the brain's reward mechanism for a more long-term, healthy mindset.

FEAR OF MISSING OUT (FOMO)

FOMO (fear of missing out) is that familiar worry that other people have better experiences than you. This fear can also be a result of the fairy-tale lives people live on social media. FOMO can leave you feeling excluded and insignificant. To remedy that, you may feel that you always have to be on the internet, checking social media and trying to be present in everything so that you don't miss out. This anxiety can have a significant negative effect on your mental health and lead to anxiety, low self-esteem, and depression. The endless measuring of your life against the ideal lives of others can leave you feeling depressed and lonely. FOMO can even disrupt sleep and lead to higher stress levels from the pressure to keep up. This anxiety tends to trigger a false high on social media, an inability to focus, and agitation. Someone suffering from FOMO may go to too many social events they don't actually enjoy, or worry more about staying connected than getting healthy.

Social media has made the fear of missing out even more pervasive. Instagram, Facebook, and TikTok routinely feature dreamscapes of people's lives—holidays, parties, milestones, everyday moments—all filtered and staged. This results in the false reality that your everyday life is less interesting than the virtual version of the life we're exposed to. Notifications, stories, and live updates all over the place keep users engaged and reinforce FOMO.

CYBERBULLYING AND ANONYMITY

Cyberbullying and anonymity are linked in the digital age when anyone with access to a computer screen can be a perpetrator of harm without direct repercussions. Anonymity is crucial in this bullying; it allows the perpetrator to operate without fear of being identified, held accountable, or subjected to punishment. Anonymity reduces the threshold for violence by making it seem remote from the victim and devoid of responsibility. Faceless people are more likely to be receptive and engage in threatening behaviors they wouldn't in person. This can be in the form of spreading gossip, posting toxic comments, threatening emails, or even making false profiles to attack targets. There are more instances of cyberbullying when it happens on a site where there are no names or no accounts to log into, like Reddit, 4chan, or comment sections on some social media sites. Anonymity makes it difficult for a victim to know who is harassing them, which makes the victim feel even more fearful, powerless, and vulnerable. This anonymity gives bullies their courage, as they are immune to the social, legal, and psychological consequences of their behavior.

Victims of cyberbullying experience a wide range of psychological side effects, such as anxiety, depression, low self-esteem, and, more serious, suicidal tendencies. Bullying can take place online all the time—harassment is a twenty-four-seven issue; it takes up room, and there is no respite for the victim. In contrast to regular bullying, which is generally confined to the school environment, cyberbullying can extend its reach into your home, which increases the severity of its effects. The anonymity of the perpetrator further magnifies the victim's feeling that they are constantly being watched or harassed, never really knowing by whom. This can result in social detachment, avoidance of internet activities, and a general feeling of insecurity.

Cyberbullying, propelled by the safety net of anonymity, is a great cyber problem. It can leave victims with irreversible scars, so it is essential that individuals, families, teachers, and platforms all come together to provide safer online spaces. The public can help tackle the tricky relationship between cyberbullying and anonymity by creating a culture of accountability, digital literacy, and support systems.

ECHO CHAMBERS AND FILTER BUBBLES

Echo chambers and filter bubbles are virtual phenomena that affect our knowledge gathering, sociability, and thought processes. They're all concepts linked directly to social media, search engines, and other online channels that cater for algorithms. This tends to confirm existing users' opinions, as well as limit exposure to different views. Echo chambers and filter bubbles promote hyperpolarization, disinformation, and diminished critical thinking.

An echo chamber is a space online where only views and facts that align with a group of beliefs can be heard. It becomes an endless loop of self-confirmation. In an echo chamber, different opinions are silenced or deliberately shut out, so the same content can be propagated and reproduced without resistance. It circulates through social media, where individuals meet like-minded people, follow certain news outlets, and consume information bearing their biases. Echo chambers can also give rise to a distortion of reality as people grow less enlightened, less accepting of difference, and more likely to believe fake or dramatic statements relevant to their narrative.

The influence is notably evident in politics, health, and social issues where echo chambers reinforce partisan schisms.

Filter bubbles arise when algorithms used by search engines of different sites such as Google, Facebook, and Twitter select what content appears to you based on your search history, clicks, likes, and shares. This customization is meant to facilitate the online experience by presenting content the user likes. But this selective sampling could lead users into a "bubble" of what they already believe while filtering out what they don't. Users may feel as if they are experiencing a lot of information when, in fact, they are only experiencing a selective part of the overall picture. This can narrow opportunities for learning, limit new knowledge, and lead to a biased view of the world.

Echo chambers and filter bubbles are part of a wider pattern of social polarization that is prominent in today's digitally linked world. Such virtual spheres reinforce the current divisions within society and prevent the exaggeration of different points of view. As a result, inaccurate information circulates quickly and unchallenged, leading to a steady loss of critical thinking. That, in turn, destabilizes public discourse, and it makes common ground more challenging. It's here that individuals have an essential role to play—actively seeking out and responding to multiple voices, and judging the voices with a critical eye. This active role is essential for building a spirit of curiosity, creating open discussion, and helping us build a more healthy and sustainable information ecosystem.

MISINFORMATION AND HARMFUL CONTENT EXPOSURE

The fake news and harmful posts on social media are becoming a huge issue because they affect mental health in large numbers. In a world where social media are the new primary outlets for news, information, and social interaction, a content that is fake, deceptive, or damaging can have major consequences for a user's mental health, leading to anxiety, stress, depression, and a misconstrued sense of reality.

Misinformation consists of false or misleading information published intentionally (disinformation) or by accident. This content spreads fast on social media because algorithms prioritize participation by focusing on dramatic, emotionally charged articles over verifiable content. Conspiracy theories, medical advice, fake pictures, and manufactured news stories are some examples. The speed and reach of false news often create confusion, anxiety, and distrust, especially in times of crisis like pandemics, elections, or natural disasters. Bad posts on social media refer to a host of negative experiences: cyberbullying, hate speech, brutality, and self-injury. Reading such material can be disruptive and traumatic in the short run. In adolescents and young adults, who are especially at risk, repeated exposure can desensitize them, make them more aggressive, and have profound emotional effects. The endless stream of disinformation, especially during a health emergency such as the COVID-19 pandemic, can amplify stress and anxiety. Deceptive information about vaccines, treatments, or emerging strains of viruses make people feel confused, nervous, and unable to rely on sources.

False narratives about lifestyles, achievement, or beauty standards foster FOMO and comparisons in which people feel inferior to online versions of their fake or hyperbolic lives. It creates a false sense of one's own worth, or lack thereof, and a constant search for validation. Threatening messages—cyberbullying, hate speech—cause loneliness and depression. The self-esteem of victims of cyberbullying reaches new lows, and those repeatedly bombarded with offensive or threatening material may develop mental health issues.

Misinformation can lead to distortions in perceptions of the world, which makes it harder for people to recognize the difference between true and false. Conspiracy theories, for example, can breed paranoia and institutional distrust, social isolation, and disconnection from the world. Video games can be highly traumatizing because many include violent content, including suicide videos for younger users. All that exposure can result in desensitization (people become unaffected by real-world pain) or hypersensitivity (people suffer extreme emotional reactions).

Specific Impact on Different Age Groups

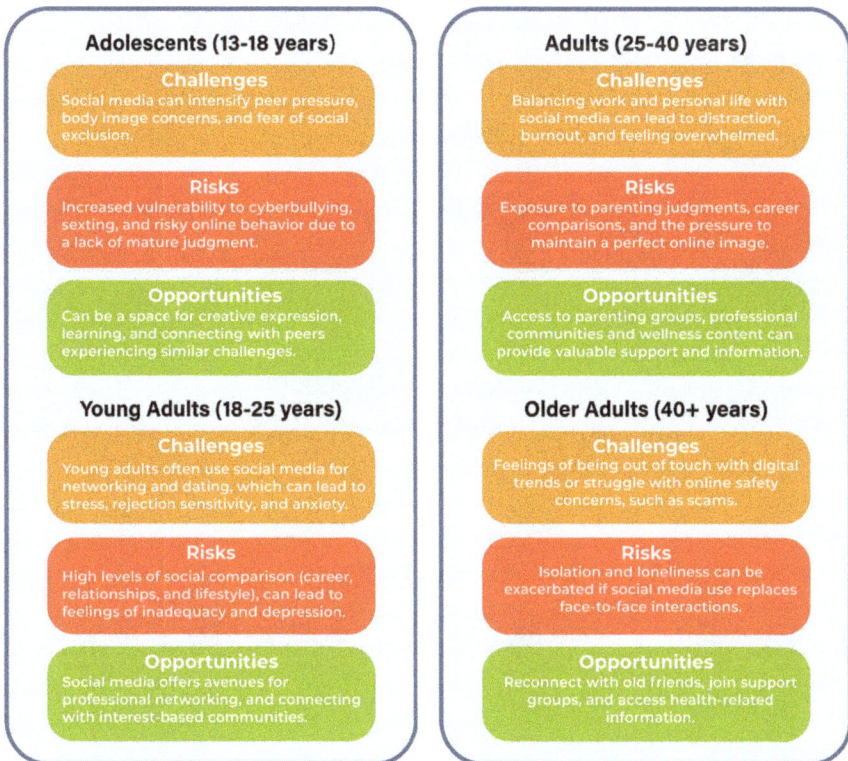

Adolescents (13-18 years)

Challenges
Social media can intensify peer pressure, body image concerns, and fear of social exclusion.

Risks
Increased vulnerability to cyberbullying, sexting, and risky online behavior due to a lack of mature judgment.

Opportunities
Can be a space for creative expression, learning, and connecting with peers experiencing similar challenges.

Young Adults (18-25 years)

Challenges
Young adults often use social media for networking and dating, which can lead to stress, rejection sensitivity, and anxiety.

Risks
High levels of social comparison (career, relationships, and lifestyle), can lead to feelings of inadequacy and depression.

Opportunities
Social media offers avenues for professional networking, and connecting with interest-based communities.

Adults (25-40 years)

Challenges
Balancing work and personal life with social media can lead to distraction, burnout, and feeling overwhelmed.

Risks
Exposure to parenting judgments, career comparisons, and the pressure to maintain a perfect online image.

Opportunities
Access to parenting groups, professional communities and wellness content can provide valuable support and information.

Older Adults (40+ years)

Challenges
Feelings of being out of touch with digital trends or struggle with online safety concerns, such as scams.

Risks
Isolation and loneliness can be exacerbated if social media use replaces face-to-face interactions.

Opportunities
Reconnect with old friends, join support groups, and access health-related information.

STRATEGIES FOR HEALTHIER SOCIAL MEDIA USE

Develop Digital Literacy and Critical Thinking

Educate Users: Understanding algorithms and recognizing misinformation can help users navigate social media more mindfully.

Critical Engagement: Question the authenticity of content and resist the urge to compare oneself to others' curated lives.

Establish Boundaries and Monitor Screen Time

Set Time Limits: Use built-in app timers or digital well-being tools to monitor and limit usage.

Designate Tech-Free Times: Prioritize offline activities during times such as meals, family time, and before bed to reduce overreliance on screens.

Curate Your Social Media Environment

Follow Positive Accounts: Surround yourself with content that inspires, educates, and uplifts rather than triggers negative feelings.

Unfollow or Mute Negative Influences: Regularly review your feed and adjust your follows to align with your current interests and mental health needs.

Engage in Meaningful Interactions

Quality Over Quantity: Focus on deep, meaningful interactions rather than superficial engagement. Engage in supportive and constructive conversations.

Avoid Toxic Debates: Steer clear of divisive or hostile discussions that can increase stress and anxiety.

Seek Professional Support When Needed

Therapy and Counseling: For those struggling with the impacts of social media on mental health, professional support can provide coping strategies and perspective.

Online Resources: Use credible mental health apps, hotlines, or digital-therapy services that offer immediate support and guidance.

Practice Mindful Social Media Use

Be Present: Avoid mindless scrolling by setting intentions for social media sessions, such as checking in with friends or learning something new.

Reflect on Your Feelings: Regularly assess how social media makes you feel. If it consistently causes distress, consider taking a break or adjusting your usage patterns.

Parental Guidance and Safety Settings

Parental Controls: For younger users, implement parental controls and monitor online interactions to ensure a safe digital environment.

Open Conversations: Encourage open dialogue between parents and children about their online experiences, fostering a supportive atmosphere.

SUMMARY AND TO-DO LIST

The impact of social media on mental health can be profoundly affected by many variables ranging from personal behavior, algorithmic structure across platforms, and social context in which such interactions take place. With careful digital education, logical boundaries, and an atmosphere of intentional and attentive consumption, consumers can remain well-adjusted and minimize any potential negative impacts of social media while still gaining useful benefits from their use. How to deal with mental health in the digital age requires an intellectually complex multidisciplinary strategy that addresses the various ways that people engage with and are shaped by the virtual worlds they inhabit.

CHAPTER V

NAVIGATING CYBERBULLYING AND ONLINE HARASSMENT

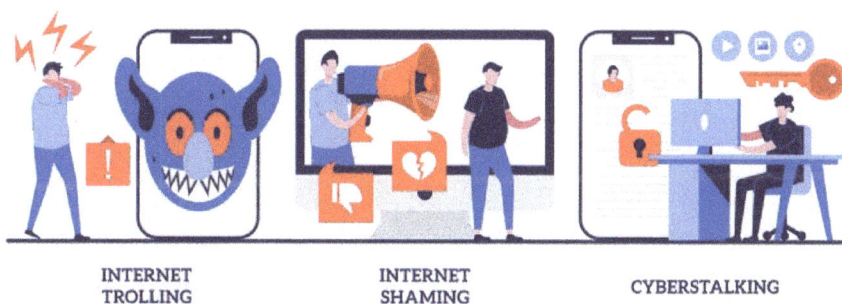

INTERNET TROLLING · INTERNET SHAMING · CYBERSTALKING

Cyberbullying is not just about bullying; it's about power and control. The key is to take back control by not engaging and seeking support.

—Carol Todd, Founder of the
Amanda Todd Legacy Society

In 2017, Bill Gates described how he and his wife, Melinda, managed their children's access to technology and social media, emphasizing setting boundaries. Gates described how he and Melinda didn't allow their children to have smartphones until the age of 14, and encouraged them to limit screen time at night until 9 o'clock in order to protect quality family time. He explained that cultivating ongoing conversations with his children about the dangers of too much social media, sleeping habits, and mental health was a central strategy to their parenting during his children's teen years. Bill Gates emphasized that his experience of how much technology could benefit education and connection, encouraged him to balance out his children's passion for technology with enabling them to use their devices mindfully. His story shows a practical approach to how tech leaders themselves promote healthy engagement, opening a case for how being a responsible parent can encourage teenagers to learn healthy digital habits.

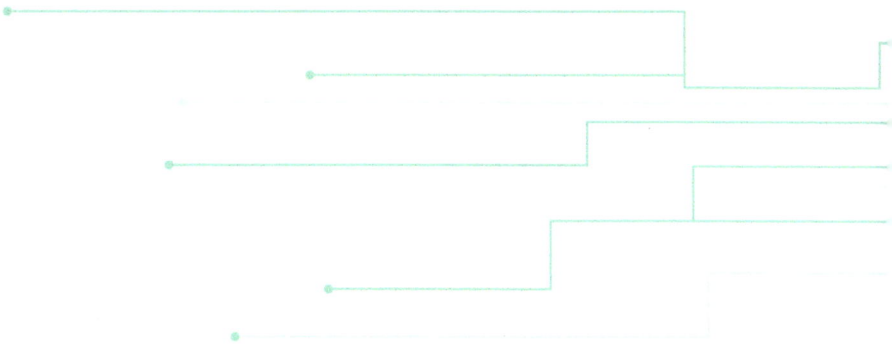

CYBERBULLYING

O nline bullying and harassment are big problems for teens on social media and other digital networks. These toxic relationships can cause profound damage to their mental health, feelings of self-worth, and sense of well-being. The Pew Research Center survey on Teens and Cyberbullying (2022) found that nearly half of all US teens aged thirteen to seventeen (46 percent) reported having experienced one or more of six types of cyberbullying. The number one problem is name-calling; 32 percent of all adolescents reported getting called vulgar names online or on cell phones. Another 22 percent have had misinformation spread about them on the internet, and 17 percent have received unsolicited erotic images. Fifteen percent have had someone ask constantly where they are and what they are doing, 10 percent have been beaten, and 7 percent have had lewd images of them circulated without their permission. Overall, 28 percent of all teens have faced at least one form of cyberbullying.

Nearly half of teens have eve experienced cyberbullying, with offensive name calling being the type most commonly reported.

% of US teens who say they have experienced cyberbullying

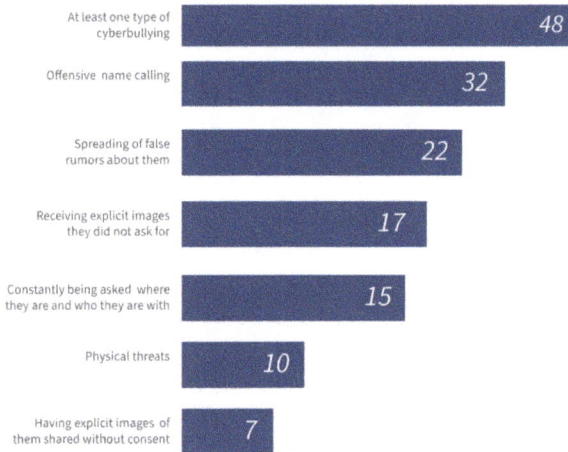

At least one type of cyberbullying	48
Offensive name calling	32
Spreading of false rumors about them	22
Receiving explicit images they did not ask for	17
Constantly being asked where they are and who they are with	15
Physical threats	10
Having explicit images of them shared without consent	7

Note: Figures may not add up to NET value.
Source: Survey of US teens conducted April - May 2022
"Teens, Social Media and Technology 2023"
PEW RESEARCH CENTER

Cyberbullying is a form of bullying done through digital technology, such as cell phones, computers, and tablets. It can be over SMS, text, mobile, social media forums, or games in which people can read, engage, or post. Cyberbullying is posting, sharing, or sending something negative, malicious, fake, or rude about someone else. This might even involve sharing something private, confidential, or humiliating. Cyberbullying can sometimes even escalate to criminal activity. In our social media and electronic communities, what we say online, whether in the form of comments, images, or other content, can be seen by a large number of people, not just our friends. All this content, good and bad, adds to our online reputation, which is accessible by anyone from potential employers and schools, to clubs and associations.

Cyberbullying damages not only the victim, but also the bullies. It is a big deal because it never goes away, and it can hurt all parties involved for the rest of their lives.

Most Common Places Where Cyberbullying Occurs

- Social media platforms, such as Facebook, Instagram, Snapchat, and TikTok
- Phone text messaging and messaging apps on mobile or tablet devices
- Instant messaging, direct messaging (on social media platforms), and online chatting over the internet
- Online forums, chat rooms, and message boards such as Reddit
- Email
- Online gaming communities

Unique Concerns

It's Persistent: Digital devices allow for continuous twenty-four-seven communication, making it challenging for cyberbullied children to seek relief.

It's Permanent: Most electronically communicated information is permanent and public. A negative online reputation, including as a result of bullying, can affect college admissions, employment, and other areas of life.

It's Hard to Notice: Cyberbullying can be difficult to recognize because it often takes place out of earshot or sight of teachers and parents.

TROLLING

Trolling is the deliberate targeting, harassing, or annoying of others by making offensive, incendiary, or infuriating comments online through social media, forums, or other forms of digital communication. Trolls, who sometimes operate under the mask of anonymity, do these things to elicit an emotional response, create tension, or just for fun. This includes everything from teasing to more serious abuse such as hate speech, threats, and misinformation.

Trolling has real implications for individuals, communities, and the internet, which it makes a hostile place. Trolling victims tend to feel stressed, anxious, and ill-protected unless the trolling is explicit or overt. These negative emotions can lead to significant mental health effects, such as depression, and internet withdrawal.

Although platforms have tried to curb trolling with moderation tools, reporting mechanisms, and tougher community policies, the problem continues to loom large in the online world. Combating trolling isn't only a matter of technical solutions; it is also about building a culture of respect and empathy online so that users can behave responsibly and ethically. The more you understand the motivation behind the trolling (attention, frustration, or group dynamics), the more you can avoid these unhealthy relationships and guard your psychological health online.

Common Trolling Tactics

Insults and Name-Calling: Using names, slurs, and insults to belittle or denigrate the victim.

Example: Posting things similar to "You're so dumb," "No one cares what you think," or using slurs to denigrate someone based on looks, intelligence, or values.

Flaming: Using a violent form of trolling in which the troll starts a heated, hostile, and usually abusive argument intended to evoke emotion.

Example: Engaging in a confrontation about controversial issues, such as politics, religion, or personal preferences, and then escalating it by using aggressive language.

Off-Topic Disruptions: Deliberately sabotaging discussions by bringing up unrelated or meaningless topics to annoy others and trash-talk.

Example: Making inane or random comments during a serious conversation to get someone else's attention or to upset someone.

Baiting: Making inflammatory comments to try to coerce others into a disagreement or battle.

Example: Saying "Nobody cares about this stuff," or "This is just dumb" and expecting it to make people mad or get a reaction.

Sarcasm and Passive-Aggressiveness: Mocking someone, saying something sarcastically, or being passive-aggressive to undermine other people.

Example: Replying with things similar to "Oh sure, because you're the expert," or "Wow, you're so creative," in a way that attempts to ridicule the other person.

Posting Misinformation: Intentionally spreading fake news, often about sensitive subjects, to mislead or upset other people.

> **Example:** Publicly circulating fake news, false numbers, or conspiracy theories to confuse and misinform people.

Ganging Up (Mob Trolling): Working in groups to get at a specific person or people and slamming them with hate speech, insults, and harangues.

> **Example:** Synchronizing attacks in which several trolls attack an individual or comment on the same post, deliberately creating a hostile environment.

Impersonation and Fake Profiles: Making fake profiles or impersonating people to cheat, deceive, or abuse.

> **Example:** Setting up an account that resembles a victim's account to circulate misinformation or engage in disputes on their behalf.

Sea-Lioning: Asking questions again and again, usually in the name of "civil" discussion, but really to wear down and anger the opposing side.

> **Example:** Requesting evidence or proof repeatedly in a manner that undermines the discussion, no matter how much there is to say.

Impact of Trolling on Teens

Emotional Distress: The psychological consequences of trolling cover a wide range, including anger, frustration, depression, and helplessness. Trolling comments are internalized by adolescents, which negatively impacts their own self-confidence and psyche.

Increased Anxiety and Depression: Persistent trolling, even if petty, can lead to anxiety, depression, and decreased sense of well-being. This is especially destructive for teenagers who are at an emotionally and socially sensitive point in their lives.

Fear of Expressing Opinions: Trolling may make it harder for teens to express themselves online, voice their opinions, or engage in conversations. A fear of being judged can lead to self-censorship and social isolation.

Disruption of Online Communities: Trolls can engulf communities and make otherwise-positive spaces hostile or uneasy. This can shut off teens from positive experiences and resources.

Normalization of Toxic Behavior: Trolling, if not properly handled, can lead to a culture of toxic norms, triggering teens to participate in or deem that behavior acceptable.

Strategies to Address and Prevent Trolling

Promote digital literacy and awareness in the following ways:

Education: Teach adolescents about trolling, its purpose, and how to identify it. Understanding that trolls look for responses helps teens to disconnect from the negativity.

Critical Thinking: Ask teens to pause and not take the bait when they hear things that might be offensive, but to discuss ideas rather than argue.

Blocking and Reporting Tools: Encourage teens to block trolls as soon as possible, end all communication, and avoid future harassing. Train teens to report trolling to platform moderators or administrators to act on inappropriate posts.

Nonengagement—Don't Feed the Trolls: Nonengagement is one of the best countermeasures to trolling. Remind teens that trolls love attention; ignoring them is typically the easiest solution.

Focus on the Good: Ask teens to direct their attention to positive and valuable interactions online instead of focusing on negative posts.

Foster resilience and self-confidence in the following ways:

Positive Support Networks: Enlist teens with a network of positive friends, family, and teachers who can be a comfort and a source of support in the face of online negativity.

Support for Mental Health: Be willing to discuss with teens how trolling has affected their mental health and seek professional assistance if necessary, particularly if trolling affects their mental health.

PLATFORM MODERATION AND COMMUNITY GUIDELINES:

Tighter Moderation: Push platforms to impose tighter community rules that discourage trolling and punish offenders.

Safe Spaces: Encourage posting in moderated forums, groups, or communities in which trolling is strictly prohibited and promptly removed.

Suggestions for Parental Involvement and Guidance:

Open Communication: Stay in contact with teens about online experiences. Be reassuring and offer tips for dealing with negative encounters.

Teaching about Privacy Settings: Help teens modify privacy settings to restrict interactions with anonymous users to prevent them from becoming target of trolls.

Use Humorous or Defusing Responses Carefully:

De-escalation: A casual or neutral response will sometimes help disarm a troll and mitigate their effects without aggravating. But do this with care, as not all trolls are predictable.

Trolling is a widespread kind of cyberbullying that can have a major impact on the mental health and safety of teens online. By educating teens, creating safe spaces, and using platform tools to stop trolls, we can help create a more secure digital world. Getting rid of trolling will take a village that includes parents, teachers, peers, and platforms to work on the principles of respect, kindness, and constructive internet interactions.

DOXING (RELEASING PRIVATE INFORMATION)

Doxing is harming someone by revealing a secret without their consent. This type of cyberbullying can be extremely damaging to the victim's safety, sense of well-being, and credibility. Doxing involves publishing information such as home addresses, phone numbers, email addresses, and job information publicly to frighten or assault the victim. It's typically used to intimidate, attack, or silence someone by threatening them. Anyone can be doxed, but generally it's activists, journalists, public figures, gamers, or anyone who has garnered online attention or criticism.

Common Methods of Doxing

Social Engineering and Phishing: Doxers employ social-engineering tactics to manipulate individuals or organizations into revealing private information. This may involve impersonating a trusted contact or using deceptive emails (phishing) to deceive victims into disclosing passwords, addresses, or other personal data.

> **Example:** Sending fake emails that look as if they are from genuine sources (like banks or social media sites) and asking the person to confirm their personal information.

Data Mining and Public Records: Doxers collect data from public records, public media, blogs, and search engines. They mine information across multiple sources to develop a profile of the target.

> **Example:** Searching someone's address, phone number, or family information on social media, work sites, or public databases.

Hacking and Password Exploitation: Doxers break into accounts to access private information directly. It can be as simple as relying on weak passwords, security vulnerabilities, or old data leaks to hack into emails, social networks, or other personal data.

> **Example:** Using passwords obtained in data breaches to steal sensitive information from an email account.

Reverse Image and Phone Number Searches: Doxers use reverse searches to find out about a photo or phone number. A simple image search, for instance, can reveal where a photo was taken or the name of someone based on a photo they shared online.

> **Example:** By uploading a profile picture to a search engine, you can find other platforms where the image appears, which may reveal additional personal information.

Crowdsourcing and Online Communities: Doxers often seek assistance from similar communities, urging others to provide information or amplify the spread of the doxed data.

> **Example:** Asking for help to identify or locate someone by posting a request on forums like 4chan, Reddit, or dark websites, and often offering rewards or recognition within the group.

Leaks from Trusted Contacts: Doxers can obtain sensitive information from individuals familiar with the target, such as former friends, partners, or disgruntled acquaintances with access to private details.

> **Example:** An ex-partner posting private messages, addresses, or other personal information to shame or threaten someone.

Impact of Doxing on Teens and Other Victims

Threats to Personal Safety

Physical Danger: Doxing can put individuals at risk of bodily harm, including stalking, harassment, and in extreme cases, swatting (falsely reporting emergencies to send police to the victim's location).

Emotional Distress: Knowing that personal information is publicly available can cause severe anxiety, fear, and paranoia, as victims worry about who might use the information against them.

Psychological Impact

Mental Health Issues: Victims of doxing often experience anxiety, depression, and PTSD-like symptoms due to the constant fear of further exposure or harassment.

Social Isolation: Fear of being targeted again can lead victims to withdraw from social interactions, both online and offline, impacting friendships, school, and work.

Reputational Damage

Public Shaming: Doxing often involves exposing private information that can embarrass or shame the victim, damaging their personal and professional reputation.

Long-Term Consequences: Once information is shared publicly, it is difficult to remove, and the impact can follow victims for years, affecting future job prospects, relationships, and community standing.

Financial Harm

Identity Theft: Exposure of sensitive information like Social Security numbers or banking details can lead to identity theft, financial fraud, and significant monetary losses.

Job Loss: Doxing can result in workplace harassment, pressure from online mobs, or employers deciding to distance themselves from controversy, which can lead to unemployment.

Protective Measures against Doxing

Enhance Privacy Settings and Minimize Personal-Information Sharing

Secure Social Media Accounts: Regularly review privacy settings on all social media platforms, ensuring that personal information is not publicly visible. Use the highest privacy settings and restrict access to trusted contacts only.

Limit Personal Details: Avoid sharing sensitive information like home addresses, phone numbers, school names, or even details that can be pieced together (like landmarks in photos) to reveal your location.

Use Strong, Unique Passwords and Two-Factor Authentication (2FA)

Password Security: Use complex, unique passwords for each account and consider using a password manager to keep track of them. Avoid using easily guessable passwords that include names, birthdays, or other apparent details.

Enable 2FA: Two-factor authentication adds an extra layer of security by requiring a second form of verification (such as a code sent to your phone) to log in, making it harder for hackers to access accounts.

Monitor Online Presence and Search for Personal Information

Regular Searches: Periodically search your name, phone number, and email address to see publicly available information. Use tools like Google Alerts to receive notifications if your information appears online.

Remove Unnecessary Data: Contact websites, forums, or data brokers to request the removal of personal information. Many platforms have processes for deleting or obscuring user data from public view.

Be Cautious with Sharing Content and Interacting Online

Be Mindful of What You Post: Consider the potential long-term consequences of what you share, including photos, check-ins, and comments that could reveal personal details.

Anonymous Browsing: To protect your identity, use pseudonyms or anonymous profiles when engaging in potentially controversial or sensitive online discussions.

Educate Teens on Safe Online Practices

Digital Literacy: Teach teens about the risks of doxing and how to protect themselves by controlling the information they share online. Encourage them to think twice before sharing personal details, even in private conversations.

Recognize Phishing Scams: Educate teens on recognizing and avoiding phishing attempts that seek to steal their personal information.

Legal Recourse and Reporting

Report Doxing to Authorities: If you are doxed, report the incident to local law enforcement, especially if threats to personal safety are involved. Some forms of doxing can be illegal, and there may be legal avenues available.

Use Platform Reporting Tools: Report doxing behavior to social media platforms to have harmful content removed and accounts suspended. Most platforms have policies against sharing personal information without consent.

Seek Support from Trusted Networks and Professionals

Reach Out: Don't face doxing alone. Contact trusted friends, family, or mental health professionals who can provide emotional support and practical advice.

Digital-Security Experts: If necessary, consult with digital-security experts to help secure your online presence, remove doxed information, and implement more robust privacy measures.

DIGITAL IMPERSONATION

Digital impersonation online involves using a person as an avatar to trick, control, or attack others. This can happen on social media, email, or other sites where someone can make a fake account or use someone else's name. The impersonation can be a threat to personal and mental health by threatening identity theft, harassment, and harm to reputation.

Types of Impersonation

Social Media Impersonation: Creating fake profiles on platforms like Instagram, Facebook, or Twitter, using someone else's name, photos, and personal details to mislead others.

Email Impersonation: Sending emails from a look-alike address and pretending to be someone else to scam recipients, spread malware, or gain sensitive information.

Catfishing: Creating a fake online persona, often on dating apps, to deceive others for financial gain, emotional manipulation, or other malicious intent.

Business Impersonation: Posing as a company representative or executive to defraud employees, partners, or customers through phishing scams or other deceptive practices.

Impact of Impersonation

Emotional Distress: Victims of impersonation often experience stress, anxiety, and emotional trauma, particularly if their personal information or reputation is damaged.

Financial Loss: Impersonators can scam individuals or businesses out of money by posing as trusted contacts, leading to significant economic losses.

Identity Theft: Impersonation can lead to stolen personal information being used for fraudulent activities such as opening accounts or making purchases.

Reputational Damage: Fake accounts can post harmful or misleading information, damaging the victim's reputation or personal relationships.

CYBERSTALKING

Cyberstalking involves persistent and unwanted monitoring or harassment of someone online. This includes frequent messaging, obsessively following the victim's online activity, or tracking their location using social media check-ins.

Cyberstalking can cause severe anxiety and fear for personal safety, leading teens to feel trapped or helpless.

SEXTORTION

Sextortion is a digital blackmail in which victims are pressured into sending pornographic images, videos, or money by threatening to divulge confidential and private data. This act generally starts with direct contact over the internet—whether via social media, dating websites, or instant messages—in which the criminal gains the trust of the victim or compromises his/her information. After snatching the compromising information, the perpetrator makes threats and terrorizes the victim.

Sextortion is a very serious crime that can result in devastating emotional, psychological, and economic harm to victims of all ages, especially teenagers and young adults who are particularly vulnerable.

How Sextortion Works

Social Engineering and Grooming: Perpetrators often pose as friendly individuals, romantic interests, or peers to gain trust. They may initially engage in casual conversations, gradually becoming flirtatious or intimate, prompting the victim to share private photos or videos.

Hacking and Unauthorized Access: Some sextortionists gain access to private devices, accounts, or webcams through hacking. By planting malware or phishing for log-in credentials, they can secretly collect explicit images or videos without the victim's knowledge.

Catfishing: Perpetrators create fake profiles on social media or dating apps, posing as someone attractive or relatable. They may manipulate the victim into sharing explicit content, which they then use as leverage for making demands.

Threats and Blackmail: Once the perpetrator has compromising material, they threaten to share it with friends, family, and others, or post it publicly unless the victim meets their demands, which can include sending more explicit content, money, or personal information.

Revenge Porn: Revenge porn refers to the nonconsensual sharing of intimate images or videos to embarrass or harm the victim.

Impact of Sextortion

Emotional and Psychological Trauma: Victims often experience intense fear, anxiety, shame, and depression. The violation of privacy and the stress of ongoing threats can severely impact mental health, leading to PTSD, withdrawal, self-harm, or suicidal thoughts.

Social and Reputational Damage: The threat of exposure can cause significant reputational harm, damaging relationships with family, friends, or colleagues. Even just the fear of exposure can be deeply distressing.

Financial Loss: Some victims are coerced into paying large sums of money to prevent their private images from being released. Unfortunately, paying does not guarantee safety, as perpetrators often continue their demands.

Loss of Trust in Online Interactions: Sextortion can cause lasting distrust in online relationships, making victims wary of forming new connections, whether personal or professional.

How to Protect Yourself from Sextortion

Limit Sharing of Personal and Intimate Content: Don't share, even with trusted individuals, explicit images or videos. Once shared, you can't control the use of that content. Avoid any individual who coerces you into sharing personal material, especially early in the relationship.

Strengthen Your Online Security: Keep account passwords unique, set two-factor authentication, and be wary of what apps and links you open. Make sure to regularly update privacy settings on social media so only trusted people can see your content and posts.

Avoid Interacting with Strangers Online: Do not trust friend requests and messages from strangers, or followers you don't know. The scammers pretend to be attractive or amiable in order to take your money. Check profiles. Don't share information about yourself with people you haven't met before.

Cover Your Webcam When Not in Use: Hackers can gain unauthorized access to your webcam without your knowledge. Keep your webcam covered or disabled when not in use to prevent unintentional recording.

Educate Yourself and Others about Sextortion: Encouraging awareness about sextortion strategies allows victims to spot warning signs in the first place. Teens should be taught the risks and encouraged to share openly about their online experiences with parents, educators, and guardians.

What to Do if You Are a Victim of Sextortion

Do Not Comply with Demands: Do not send additional content, money, or any personal information. Rather than resolving the situation, compliance often leads to more threats and demands.

Report the Incident: Report the perpetrator to the platform on which the interaction took place and to local law enforcement. Most social media and online platforms have procedures to handle such threats and can assist in removing content.

Seek Support: Reach out to trusted friends, family, or professional counselors for emotional support. Organizations like the National Center for Missing and Exploited Children, Cyber Civil Rights Initiative, and local hotlines can provide guidance and resources.

Preserve Evidence: Save screenshots, messages, and any other evidence of the threats or blackmail attempts. This information is valuable for law enforcement and platform investigations.

Consult Cybersecurity Professionals: If your accounts or devices were compromised, seek help from cybersecurity experts who can secure your data, remove malware, and restore your digital security.

BODY-SHAMING AND SLUT-SHAMING

Body-shaming and slut-shaming are harmful social practices whereby someone is criticized or ridiculed for how they look or feel about sexuality. These behaviors can have devastating emotional, psychological, and social consequences, especially among adolescents and young adults who are at the highest risk from society's pressures and stigmatization.

Common Forms of Body-Shaming and Slut-Shaming

Weight Shaming: Criticizing someone for being too thin, overweight, or not fitting conventional body standards.

Appearance-Based Insults: Mocking someone for specific physical features, such as acne, stretch marks, or body hair.

Comparisons to Unrealistic Standards: Comparing individuals to edited or idealized images seen in media and advertising, which leads to feelings of inadequacy.

Shaming Based on Clothing Choices: Criticizing someone for wearing clothes that don't fit traditional beauty norms, whether because they are too revealing or not flattering.

Judging Sexual Behavior: Condemning someone for having multiple partners, engaging in casual sex, or discussing their sexual experiences openly.

Blaming Victims of Sexual Harassment or Assault: Suggesting that someone "asked for it" based on their behavior, appearance, or previous sexual history.

Mental Health Issues: Body-shaming can lead to low self-esteem, anxiety, depression, eating disorders, and even suicidal thoughts.

Body Dysmorphia: A distorted perception of one's own body and obsessing over perceived flaws; this is often exacerbated by external criticism.

Social Withdrawal: Victims of body-shaming may withdraw from social interactions, thereby avoiding situations where they feel they will be judged or exposed, like swimming pools or gyms.

Negative Self-Image: Internalizing critical comments can lead to a long-term negative self-image, affecting how individuals perceive and value themselves.

Damaged Reputation: Slut-shaming can severely damage a person's reputation, affecting their relationships, academic or professional opportunities, and how they are perceived by peers.

PREVENTION AND COPING STRATEGIES FOR TEENS

It takes parents, educators, peers, and the platforms working in partnership to solve the widespread problem of online bullying and harassment. You should teach teens at an early age, with detailed information, about internet harassment such as cyberbullying, online shaming, doxing, and trolling. By providing them with the options of reporting, blocking, and requesting the assistance needed to handle these challenges, we will be able to make the internet a safer, better place. That model promotes healthy digital relationships and enhanced well-being among youth.

Smart Tips

Online Harassment Coping Strategies

1. **BECOME EDUCATED AND BE AWARE**

2. **ENCOURAGE OPEN COMMUNICATIONS**

3. **PROMOTE DIGITAL LITERACY**

4. **USE REPORTING AND BLOCKING TOOLS**

5. **SEEK PROFESSIONAL SUPPORT**

CHAPTER VI

DIGITAL SAFETY 101

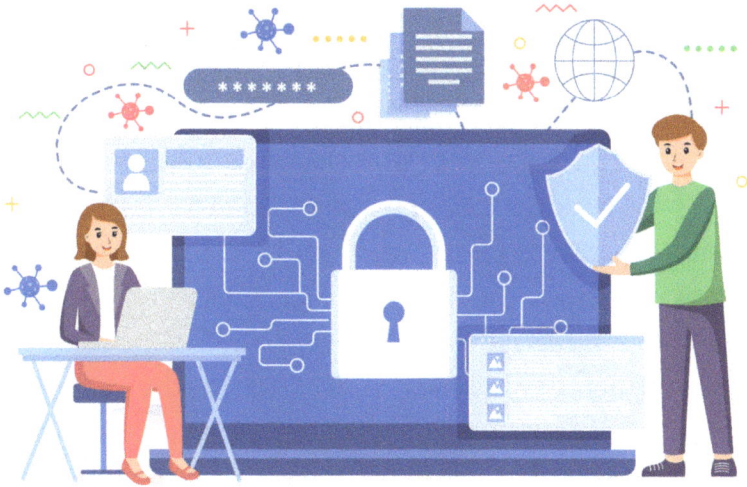

In 2019, the cofounder of Twitter, Jack Dorsey, was among the most prominent tech-industry figures to be afflicted by a digital security breach. Well-known as a cryptocurrency enthusiast, Dorsey's Twitter account was hacked by a group of hackers who used his handle to spread racist and Islamophobic material, and promote the hackers' site. The attack pointed to an unusual part of the data theft—the hacker obtained Dorsey's account via a process called SIM swapping. The hackers took someone else's phone number and used it to reset Dorsey's Twitter password and open his account. Twitter users and others worldwide were reminded of just how vulnerable they are.

If the founder of one of the largest social media companies in the world could have his account hijacked by hackers, the need to protect your digital data beyond using passwords alone became apparent. Much was made of the hack, with Twitter and other companies tweeting reminders about the need to safeguard accounts through multifactor authentication, as well as guidance about understanding SIM swapping. The Big Tech Hack highlighted that digital safety remains an issue for everyone, regardless of your knowledge or status as a tech developer versus just a regular user.

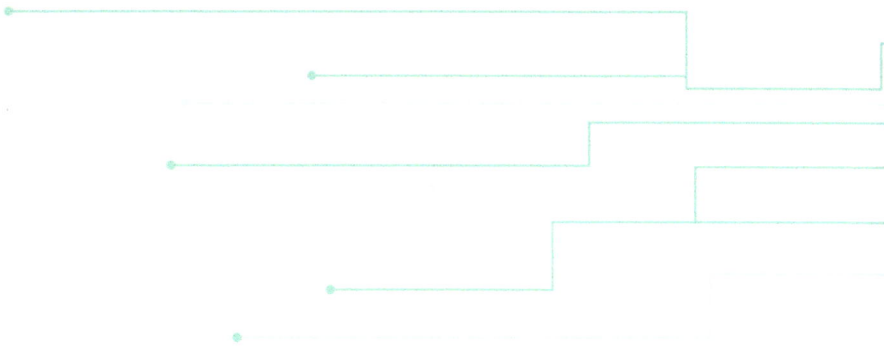

Digital safety refers to the methods and measures adopted to maintain your privacy, data, and health while engaging in the digital realm. As technology increasingly permeates our everyday life, you need to protect your data and online presence to ensure against hackers, phishing, identity theft, and cyberbullying. Digital safety covers a range of topics, such as creating unique passwords, setting up two-factor authentication (2FA), and updating devices and software to prevent security issues. It's also essential to remain on the alert for phishing scams—attempts to take sensitive data by sending forged emails, text messages, or landing pages.

You can keep your social media privacy protected by setting your options, restricting your content, and keeping your digital footprint safe from hackers and exploitation. Additionally, use of secure networks, especially when working with sensitive data, and virtual private networks (VPNs) when connected to public Wi-Fi are other practices that can help you protect your web-browsing habits.

Digital safety also includes identifying and reporting cyberbullying, harassment, and other harmful online behaviors in order to ensure a respectful and safe space. It

is important to navigate the internet safely, to keep your data secure, and to provide an enjoyable and safe online experience for yourself and others.

PRIVACY SETTINGS

Privacy settings on social media are vital to limit who sees what you post, who can interact with you, and who can view your information. If you use these options wisely, you can maintain privacy, avoid unwelcome content, and become more safe online. Here's how to use privacy settings correctly on social media:

Set Your Profile to Private: Be sure to set your account to private. If you have a private profile, only verified followers or friends will be able to see your posts and details. This is necessary because setting your account to private allows you to impose rules about who can access your post, thereby restricting it to people you trust.

Limit Who Can Find You: For online platforms, you should be careful about who can find your profile. This includes those who look you up using your email address or phone number. Facebook, Instagram, and other social media platforms have privacy settings you can adjust to decide how searchable your profile is. Changing these options will help you avoid unwanted contacts or strangers. It allows you to be more in control of who finds you and contacts you. And you can choose to limit who can see your posts, giving yourself more control over what happens online and how you're viewed.

Control Who Can See Your Posts and Stories: When posting on social media, you can use the post settings to control the visibility of each individual post or story. The options often include Public, Friends, Close Friends, or Custom; each of these choices are linked to a contact list of your making. This feature allows you to share specific content with selected audiences based on your preferences, thereby safeguarding your privacy and ensuring that sensitive information is only shared with the intended audience.

Manage Your Friends and Followers: Be sure to keep checking your social media friends/followers list on a regular basis and unfollow those whom you don't know or trust. Utilize the options to manually approve new followers rather than auto-approving them. That extra precaution means that only people you're comfortable sharing your posts and information with will see them, maintaining you online privacy and safe.

Adjust Tagging and Mentions Settings: To enhance your privacy and protect your reputation, consider adjusting your settings to require your approval before others can tag you in photos, posts, or mentions. Doing this, you'll also have control over who can tag or mention you, which can help prevent any unwanted associations with content that might compromise your privacy or professional image.

Review Location-Sharing Settings: To enhance your personal safety, consider taking the following measures regarding location sharing: Turn off location services on your device or limit location sharing in your social media posts, stories, and check-ins. If possible, disable real-time location sharing unless it is absolutely necessary. These steps will protect your whereabouts and prevent strangers from knowing your location, thus enhancing your personal safety.

Control Who Can Comment or Message You: To enhance your online safety and reduce exposure to cyberbullying, spam, and unwanted interactions, you can adjust your social media account settings to control who can comment on your posts or message you directly. You can choose to limit these interactions to your friends only or completely turn off comments. By doing so, you can create a more secure and inviting online environment.

Review Your Privacy Settings Regularly: To safeguard your privacy, it's important to make a habit of frequently reviewing and adjusting your privacy settings, particularly following platform updates or modifications to privacy policies. By doing so, you can ensure that your settings remain current and that they effectively cater to your privacy requirements as the landscape of social media continues to change and evolve.

Limit Access to Your Personal Information: Be careful what you put on the internet. Don't post intimate information like your birthday, home address, phone number, and school or office information. Use privacy settings to make sure this is only shown to the people you want it to be seen by and only share with people you trust. By following these steps, you can avoid a lot of the identity theft, stalking, and other potential risks that come with sharing too much information on the internet.

Use Two-Factor Authentication (2FA): Setting up two-factor authentication (2FA) is an additional security measure to help secure your account. When 2FA is enabled, besides typing in your password, you will be asked to provide a second level of authentication—for example, a unique code delivered to your phone or generated by an authentication app. This second verification step makes it much less likely that someone will ever get into your account without the second verification. By adding 2FA, you're protecting your account and making it more resistant to unauthorized access.

With the right privacy settings on social media, you will have more control over your life online, you will be able to protect your data, and you will have a safer and more enjoyable experience. The key to maintaining digital privacy is regularly revisiting your settings and being alert to what you are sharing.

RECOGNIZING SCAMS, PHISHING, AND PREDATORY BEHAVIORS ONLINE

Detecting scams, phishing attempts, and predatory activities is crucial for safeguarding your data and ensuring digital safety. Hackers and predators use a variety of methods to trick, cheat, or abuse unsuspecting users—usually young people and other weaker groups. Here's how to recognize these dangers and remain safe online.

Recognizing Scams

Unsolicited Messages or Offers: Scammers often send unsolicited messages promising easy money, prizes, or exclusive offers. If it sounds too good to be true, it probably is.

Red Flags: Messages from unknown contacts, suspicious links, requests for personal information, or urgent language pushing you to act quickly.

Requests for Personal or Financial Information: Scammers may pose as legitimate companies or individuals asking for sensitive information, like credit card numbers, passwords, or Social Security numbers.

> **Red Flags:** Requests for sensitive information via email, text, or social media, especially if the communication seems unprofessional or is riddled with spelling errors.

Impersonation of Trusted Entities: Scammers often impersonate trusted companies, friends, or even family members to gain your trust.

> **Red Flags:** Misspellings of company names, slight alterations in email addresses, and urgent requests that seem out of character.

Recognizing Phishing Attempts

Suspicious Emails and Messages: Phishing emails or messages attempt to trick you into clicking on malicious links or downloading harmful attachments often disguised as urgent alerts, invoices, or account updates.

> **Red Flags:** Emails from unknown senders, generic greetings such as "Dear Customer," mismatched URLs, and links that don't match the official website.

Fake Log-in Pages: Phishing scams often direct you to fake log-in pages that look like legitimate sites (for example, bank or social media log-ins) to steal your credentials.

> **Red Flags:** URLs that are slightly misspelled, sites that don't look quite right, and requests for information that a legitimate site wouldn't typically ask for.

Social Media Phishing: Scammers may use direct messages or fake profiles on social media to lure you into providing personal information or clicking malicious links.

> **Red Flags:** Unfamiliar accounts sending friend requests, strange messages from known contacts, or links that don't seem relevant.

Recognizing Predatory Behaviors

Grooming Tactics: Predators often use grooming techniques to gain a victim's trust, gradually manipulating them into sharing personal information, photos, or engaging in inappropriate activities.

> **Red Flags:** Excessive flattery, requests for secrecy, age-inappropriate conversations, and pushing for personal or private information.

Attempts to Isolate or Control: Predators may try to isolate you from friends or family by encouraging secrecy or exclusive online contact.

> **Red Flags:** Encouraging you to keep conversations private, requesting private chats or video calls, or becoming upset if you talk to others.

Uncomfortable or Inappropriate Interactions: Any behavior that feels off—such as asking for photos, pushing boundaries, or making you feel pressured—can be a sign of predatory intent.

> **Red Flags:** Requests for personal photos, persistent or overly personal questions, or any form of coercion.

SUMMARY AND TO-DO LIST

If you want to be safe online, you have to know the signs of scamming, phishing, and predatory activity. Scammers and cybercriminals are not above attempting to coerce you into giving out your personal information or committing a financial crime. If you're proactive, and if you're educated about common scams—fake emails, websites, unwanted phone calls—you can better recognize and dodge the threat. Additionally, by taking preventive measures—like using unique and strong passwords, implementing two-factor authentication, and upgrading your security tools—you will also be more secure on the internet. By staying alert and vigilant, you can protect your data and maintain a safe online identity.

Smart Tips

How to Protect Yourself Online

1. VERIFY BEFORE YOU TRUST

2. NEVER SHARE PERSONAL INFORMATION

3. AVOID CLICKING ON SUSPICIOUS LINKS

4. USE STRONG SECURITY MEASURES

5. TRUST YOUR INSTINCTS

CHAPTER VII

MINDFUL SOCIAL MEDIA USE

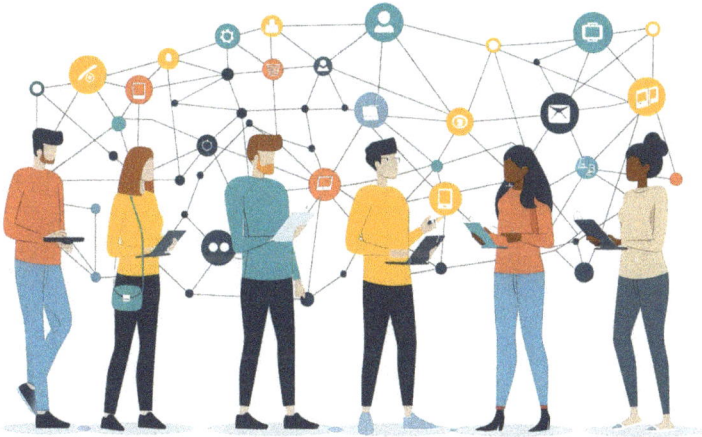

It's not about spending less time on social media, but spending better time. Curate your feed to support your well-being, not detract from it.

—Emma Watson, Actress and Activist

When the American actress Demi Lovato announced in 2019 that she was stepping off Instagram and Twitter for her mental health, many of her fans recognized that this symbolized mindful digital citizenship. The star was very open about personal insecurities and issues (including addiction, body image, and mental health) and was often honest on social media with fans. But, in interviews, she revealed that the constant exposure to negative comments and the pressures of posting regularly was exhausting her and making it hard to sustain a positive view of herself online. In a revealing statement, Lovato said that she enjoyed the connection with her fans, but she felt she needed to put herself first, over her work. She told W magazine: "I'm traveling so much, playing shows, meeting friends, but also I'm constantly on my phone, and it can be really draining and toxic."

She expressed a clear view on positivity online and a call for more thoughtfulness about the platforms we engage with: "There's no shame in stepping away from Instagram or Twitter for your mental health." Lovato's case is one of many stories demonstrating that digital citizenship is not just about being visible on the internet, but rather it's about having presence and mindful uses of digital technology, such as exiting and entering our apps thoughtfully.

Mindful social media is all about being deliberate, mindful, and balanced in your digital interactions to keep your mental health safe and online experiences positive. Because social media is a huge part of our lives, there's no excuse for mindless scrolling, comparisons, or negative interactions that can undermine your self-worth, work ethic, and mental well-being. When you use social media mindfully, you take charge of your online behaviors, and social media becomes a more productive, positive force in your life.

Being mindful starts with setting clear goals for how you use social media. Rather than opening apps randomly simply because you're in the habit of it, consider why you're going online in the first place—whether it's to share with friends, read up on something, or just chill. By limiting time and taking frequent breaks, you can prevent overload and minimize the chances of burnout, anxiety, or being overwhelmed.

Organizing your feed to include accounts that motivate, teach, or entertain, and unfollowing those that elicit negative reactions, is another important step in mindful usage. Be positive by making comments that are unbiased, sharing valuable information, and not getting into a web fight or toxic interaction. Remember, too, that social media can be a highlight reel of someone else's life, so don't set unrealistic expectations.

Lastly, think about your emotional engagement on social media. If it's impacting your mood or your self-worth, step back and recheck how engaged you are. Conscious social media is about having the right balance that will make your life better, foster real connections, and improve your mental health. If you are responsible and mindful of what you do online, then you will develop a more positive relationship with social media.

Why Mindful Social Media Use Matters for Teens

Protects Mental Health: Mindful use helps teens manage the anxiety, depression, and stress associated with excessive or negative social media interactions. By intentionally using social media, teens can minimize exposure to harmful content and cultivate a healthier online environment.

Enhances Focus and Academic Performance: Reducing mindless scrolling and setting boundaries around social media use can help teens focus better on schoolwork, improve attention spans, and enhance overall productivity.

Promotes Positive Relationships: Mindful engagement encourages teens to prioritize quality over quantity in their interactions, fostering deeper, more profound connections, rather than superficial exchanges.

Builds Resilience and Digital Literacy: By being aware of how social media impacts their thoughts, emotions, and behaviors, teens can develop critical-thinking skills and resilience, helping them navigate digital spaces more safely.

Encourages Healthy Self-Expression: Mindfulness allows teens to express themselves authentically without succumbing to the pressures of social validation, thereby helping them build a positive self-image.

CHALLENGES TO MINDFUL SOCIAL MEDIA USE FOR TEENS

Social Validation and Peer Pressure: The desire for likes, comments, and followers can lead to addictive behavior and constant comparison with others, both of which undermine self-esteem and promote anxiety.

FOMO (Fear of Missing Out): FOMO drives teens to stay constantly connected, leading to compulsive checking of feeds and notifications to avoid missing out on social events, trends, or updates from friends.

Algorithm-Driven Content Consumption: Social media platforms are designed to keep users engaged through algorithm-driven feeds that prioritize highly engaging content, often pulling teens into endless scrolling sessions.

Exposure to Negative or Inappropriate Content: Teens may encounter cyberbullying, hate speech, or unrealistic beauty standards, all of which can negatively impact their mental health and self-image.

STRATEGIES FOR PROMOTING MINDFUL SOCIAL MEDIA USE AMONG TEENS

Promoting mindful social media use among teens involves encouraging intentional, balanced, and positive engagement with digital platforms. Here are some key strategies:

Pause & Reflect

Teach to pause and consider before posting or responding to content.

Helps prevent impulsive actions that could lead to regret or conflict.

Give Positive Feedback

Encourage teens to follow uplifting and educational accounts.

Contributes to a healthier mindset and reduces impact of harmful content.

Set Intentions

Encourage teens to ask themselves why they are logging on before opening an app.

Helps teens differentiate between productive use and mindless scrolling

Create Balance

Encourage teens to balance social media use with offline activies.

Balancing online and offline activies is essential for avoidning dependancy and digital validation.

Limit Screen Time

built-in screen time trackers on phones or apps and set daily time limits for social media use.

Setting boundaries helps manage time and reduces negative impacts on mental health.

Screen Breaks

Designate specific time of the day that are socail-media free.

Helps recharge, improves quality of sleep and develops healthier routines.

Manage Notifications

Turn off non-essential notifications or set specific times to check updates.

Helps teens stay focused on present tasks and reduces the compulsion to constantly check their phones.

Meaningful Interactions

Encourage teens to engage in genuine conversations rather than chasing likes.

Meaningful interactions build deeper connections and promote a sense of belonging.

Seek Support

Encourage open communications about their online experiences.

Supportive environment ensure teens feel comfortable discussing their digital struggles.

Offline Socialization

Emphasize the value of face-to-face interactions over online-only friendships.

Offline relationships helps counterbalance the sometimes shallow nature of online connections.

SUMMARY AND TO-DO LIST

Being mindful of the perils of social media is good for teenagers. Adolescents must be given the tools to regulate their online presence in ways that will protect and enhance their mental health, self-discovery, and well-being. Teens can do this by setting boundaries explicitly, by being mindful of their interactions, and by engaging in a healthy manner on social media. Parents, teachers, and others within our communities must make the effort to lead teens toward adopting healthy social media practices and fostering a balanced digital lifestyle.

Smart Tips

Mindful Social Media Use

1. SET INTENTIONS BEFORE LOGGING ON

2. LIMIT NOTIFICATIONS TO REDUCE DISTRACTIONS

3. REFLECT YOUR VALUES IN WHO YOU FOLLOW

4. ENGAGE WITH PURPOSE, NOT IMPULSE

5. TAKE REGULAR BREAKS TO RESET

CHAPTER VIII

COMMUNITY ENGAGEMENT IN SOCIAL MEDIA SAFETY AND WELLNESS FOR TEENS

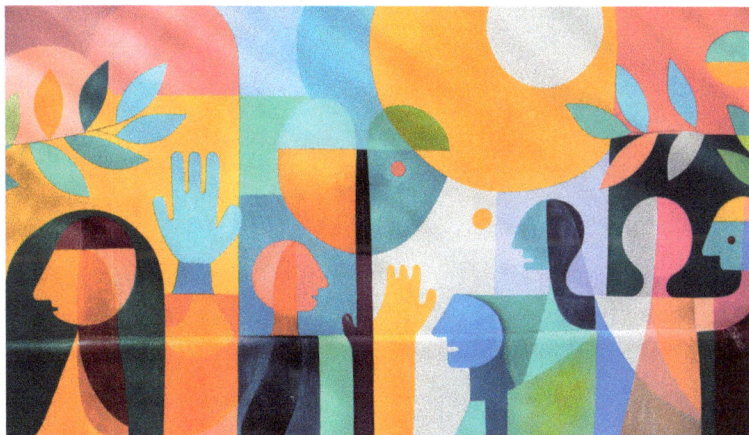

It takes a village to support a teen's mental health. Schools, parents, and peers all play a role in creating a network of care and understanding.

—Simone Biles, Olympic Gymnast
and Mental Health Advocate

Pop star Ariana Grande initiated a community of care focused on teens' mental health through her own social media in 2018. After a heartbreaking bombing at the Manchester Arena the previous year, and just before releasing her newest album, Sweetener, Ariana shifted her digital presence to one of hope, encouragement, and support. Her social feed consisted of self-love and mental health messages, bringing many millions of young fans together in a community of care and vocal activism. She frequently posted about taking care of herself, seeing a therapist, and regularly engaging with her fans to encourage questions. Teens participating in this online social media community were inspired to care for their minds and ask for help when needed. There was a beautiful snowball effect to all of this wellness posting. The posts inspired conversations about challenges and good days, and Ariana's words generated waves of positivity within the community that surrounded her. She showed genuine support and "liked" the teenagers' positive posts and responses, bringing light into the world and holding up others who were raising awareness of their feelings.

In 2021, actress Jennifer Garner became vocal about parental involvement in their kids' social media use, sharing how she tackles this with her kids, twin teenagers. In interviews, she was candid about how she turned off devices at mealtimes and closely watched the screen time of her teenagers while making an effort to engage in their digital life, sitting with them and talking about what they liked, whom they were following, what content was troubling them, how they felt, or what they felt others could do to intervene when someone was not feeling well. She also shared how she instigated family "digital detox" days at least once a month, a day during which everyone unplugged and did something together offline. This way, she stayed involved but didn't cross over into an overinvolved approach.

Jennifer created an atmosphere of being able to engage in conversations around the use of social media in a healthy way, without being alarmist, recognizing both the vital role of technology plays for mental health and well-being and the fact that it needs to be moderated. She stressed the importance of parental influence to help teens develop a healthy relationship with the online world—where their mental health is paramount.

I t's important to include the community in the process of ensuring teens' social media safety and well-being. By including parents, educators, therapists, and others, the community creates a positive context for digital well-being and shields teens from the harms of social media.

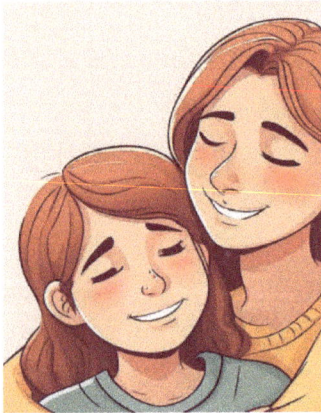

ROLE OF PARENTS AND GUARDIANS

Parents and guardians are often the first line of defense in guiding teens toward safe and healthy social media use. Their involvement can help teens navigate the complexities of digital spaces.

Using Open Communication

Importance: Encouraging open, nonjudgmental conversations about social media use helps teens feel supported and understood. Discussing online experiences, both positive and negative, can reduce feelings of isolation and anxiety.

Strategies: Regularly ask teens about their favorite platforms, whom they interact with, and how specific content makes them feel. Use these conversations to guide teens in identifying what is healthy or potentially harmful.

Setting Boundaries and Digital Etiquette

Importance: Establishing rules around screen time, privacy settings, and appropriate online behavior can create a safer digital environment.

Strategies: Work with teens to set realistic screen-time limits, monitor app usage, and use parental controls where appropriate. Teach digital etiquette, including how to handle cyberbullying, avoid oversharing, and respecting others online.

Modeling Healthy Behavior

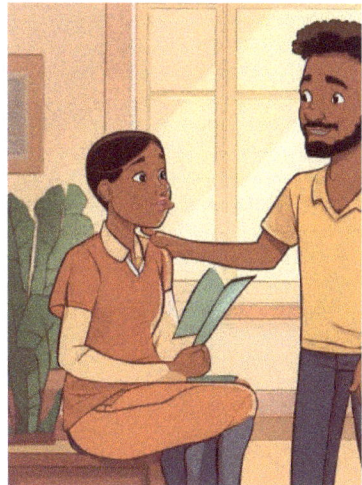

Importance: Teenagers often mimic the online behavior of adults in their lives. Parents can set a positive example by modeling mindful and balanced social media use.

Strategies: Demonstrate responsible use, such as not being constantly on your phone during family time, avoiding negative online interactions, and taking regular breaks from social media.

INVOLVEMENT OF EDUCATORS AND SCHOOLS

Schools are pivotal in shaping teens' understanding of digital safety and wellness, and integrating these lessons into the broader educational framework.

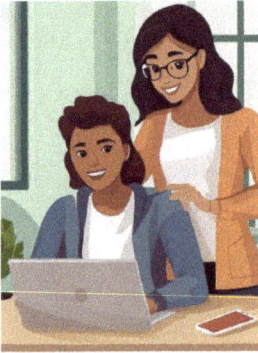

Digital Literacy Programs

Importance: Educating teens about digital literacy, online privacy, and the impact of social media on mental health empowers them to make informed decisions.

Strategies: Incorporate digital literacy into the curriculum, teaching students about recognizing misinformation, understanding algorithms, and protecting their digital footprints. Use real-life examples and interactive activities to keep lessons engaging.

Workshops and Assemblies on Social Media Safety

Importance: Hosting workshops or assemblies on social media safety can provide valuable information and strategies directly to students.

Strategies: Partner with mental health professionals, social media experts, or digital-safety organizations to conduct sessions on cyberbullying prevention, managing screen time, and promoting mental wellness online.

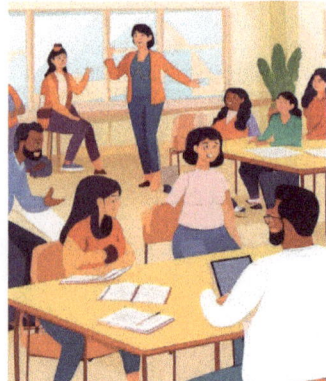

Peer-Mentorship Programs

Importance: Peer influence is powerful among teens. Peer-mentorship programs can leverage this dynamic to promote positive online behaviors.

Strategies: Train older students or student leaders to mentor younger peers on safe social media use, provide relatable guidance, and create a supportive school culture.

ROLE OF MENTAL HEALTH PROFESSIONALS AND COMMUNITY ORGANIZATIONS

Mental health professionals and community organizations are crucial in supporting teens' mental wellness and social media safety.

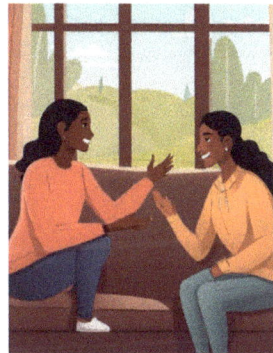

Counseling and Support Services

Importance: Access to counseling services can help teens navigate the emotional impacts of social media, such as anxiety, depression, or cyberbullying.

Strategies: Schools and community centers should provide access to mental health professionals who can offer one-on-one counseling, group-therapy sessions, or workshops focused on coping strategies and resilience.

Community Programs and Workshops

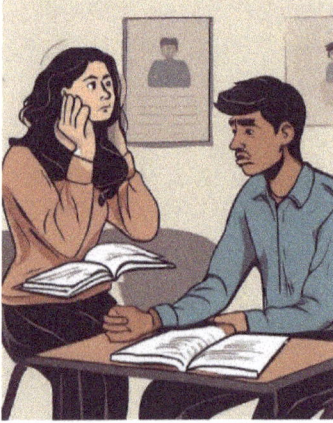

Importance: Community programs can offer resources and education for teens and parents, helping them better understand the digital landscape.

Strategies: Organize workshops on social media safety, mental health, and digital well-being. These programs can cover topics such as digital detox, managing online stress, and building self-esteem outside social validation.

Online Safety Campaigns

Importance: Public-awareness campaigns can reach a broad audience, promoting safe and healthy social media use on a larger scale.

Strategies: Community organizations can collaborate with schools, local governments, and tech companies to create campaigns highlighting the importance of online safety, privacy, and mental wellness.

ENGAGING TEENS AS ACTIVE PARTICIPANTS

Empowering teens to take an active role in their social media safety and wellness fosters a sense of responsibility and self-awareness.

Youth-Led Initiatives

Importance: Allowing teens to lead initiatives related to social media safety helps them develop leadership skills and advocate for their peers.

Strategies: Support the creation of teen-led clubs or groups that focus on digital wellness. These groups can run awareness campaigns, create supportive content, or host discussions on social media experiences.

Teen Involvement in Content Creation

Importance: Teens are more likely to respond to content created by their peers. Involving them in creating educational videos, social media posts, or digital guides can make the messages more relatable.

Strategies: Encourage teens to produce content that promotes positive online behavior, such as videos on managing privacy settings or graphics on coping with online stress.

Feedback and Listening Sessions

Importance: Listening to teens about their concerns and experiences with social media provides valuable insights and helps adults address the real issues teens face.

Strategies: Host regular listening sessions or feedback forums in which teens can openly share their thoughts about social media. Use this feedback to adapt safety and wellness initiatives to meet their needs better.

LEVERAGING TECHNOLOGY AND ONLINE TOOLS

Technology can help create safer and healthier online experiences for teens through monitoring, education, and engagement.

Safety Tools and Apps

Importance: Numerous apps and tools help monitor social media activity, block harmful content, and support mental health.

Strategies: Educate teens and parents about apps that track screen time, filter content, or provide access to mental health resources, such as Headspace for mindfulness or Bark for social media monitoring.

Safe Online Spaces

Importance: Digital platforms can partner with communities to create safe spaces where teens can engage without fear of harassment or negative interactions.

Strategies: Promote moderated online communities or apps specifically designed for teen wellness, such as forums to discuss mental health topics in a safe environment.

COLLABORATIVE EFFORTS WITH SOCIAL MEDIA PLATFORMS

Social media companies can play a proactive role by working with communities to enhance platform safety features and promote wellness.

Safety Features and Reporting Tools

Importance: Platforms like Instagram, TikTok, and YouTube have developed tools to help manage screen time, report harmful content, and limit unwanted interactions.

Strategies: Educate teens on using these tools effectively and encourage platforms to continuously update their safety measures in response to emerging risks.

Mental Health Awareness Campaigns

Importance: Social media platforms can use their reach to promote mental health awareness, providing resources directly within the app.

Strategies: Collaborate with mental health organizations to run in-app campaigns during Mental Health Awareness Month or other relevant periods, offering tips on managing online stress or where to seek help.

SUMMARY AND TO-DO LIST

Communal involvement plays an important role in social media safety and teens' mental health. Developing a holistic support network involves partnering with parents, teachers, mental health care providers, and teens. This all-inclusive model enables our youth to navigate the social media landscape safely and securely. By bringing different stakeholders together, we can ensure teens are equipped with the skills, information, and resources to make informed decisions when engaging with digital technology. This partnership is critical to ensuring that adolescents maintain a healthy relationship with social media.

Smart Tips

Community Engagement

1. CREATE SAFE AND INCLUSIVE SPACES

2. OFFER MENTAL HEALTH RESOURCES

3. INVOLVE TEENS IN PLANNING

4. PROMOTE PEER SUPPORT NETWORKS

5. UTILIZE DIGITAL TOOLS AND PLATFORMS

CHAPTER IX

BUILDING RESILIENCE
AND SELF-CARE PRACTICES

STEPS TO MENTAL HEALTH

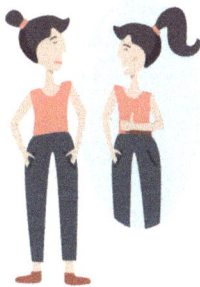

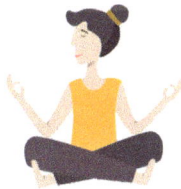

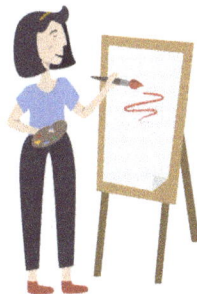

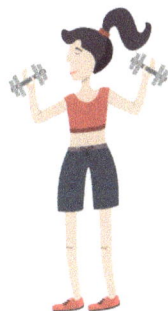

SELF-ACCEPTANCE

RELAX

GET CREATIVE

STAY ACTIVE

*Building resilience in the digital age means knowing
when to step back, unplug, and prioritize your
mental health over the endless scroll.*

—Dr. Brené Brown, Author and Researcher

In 2021, singer Shawn Mendes spoke out about his mental self-care practices and how they shaped his well-being as an adolescent. He described having anxiety, which led to overweening behavior and fear, and how he countered it with his mind through meditation, journaling, and daily affirmations. He also shared that seeking help through therapy supported him in dealing with his problems; it taught him the skills he needed to cope in a healthier way.

His testimony's intention was to encourage teenagers to care for themselves and seek support when needed: The road to better mental health doesn't have to be miserable. While we're often told to push through challenges, to be stronger, resilient internet entrepreneurs like Elon Musk are pushing a different narrative, which is to avoid pain at all costs. But mental resilience isn't an absence of pain; it is the use of resources that equip us to face it.

Prince Harry highlighted in 2020 the importance of resilience and self-care to mental health, especially among young people. In his consultancy for the non-profit group Heads Together, Harry stressed the need to enable teenagers to discuss their mental health issues without shame. He said that his own approach to resilience started by consulting with professionals and putting exercise, nature, and mindfulness into his daily schedule. Prince Harry added that asking for support is not a sign of weakness, but a powerful healing act. His open-mindedness and attempts to normalize mental health discourse inspired many teens struggling in similar ways. Through his messages of open dialogue and self-care, Prince Harry vowed to make the world a place where youth feel free to invest in their own mental health and learn the skills to cope with challenges in life.

The power of self-care has never been more needed in our busy digital society. When our lifestyle is increasingly driven by technology, it can be hard to balance our minds and bodies, especially when we are so consumed by screens and the internet. Breathing exercises, journaling, and mindfulness apps are all accessible ways to finding peace within and relieving stress. Understanding how to manage online negative relationships and tension between the virtual and physical realms can help one live a better life.

BREATHING EXERCISES: SIMPLE YET POWERFUL SELF-CARE

Breathing exercises are one of the simplest, most efficient forms of self-care that you can do. They involve intentional deep breathing that will relieve stress, increase attention spans, and promote relaxation. Breathing activities engage the parasympathetic nervous system, which quiets the body's stress response. This is especially useful when you are feeling anxious or overwhelmed. Just a few minutes of concentrated breathing can make you feel in control and calm.

A popular technique is diaphragmatic breathing, or belly breathing. It is the process of taking a deep breath through the nose and stretching the diaphragm, then slowly exhaling through the mouth. This technique increases oxygenation, slows down heart rate, and allows relaxation.

The 4–7–8 breathing technique is also a good one; it consists of breathing for four seconds, holding your breath for seven seconds, and then breathing out for eight seconds. This practice is relaxing and recommended for calming and enhancing sleep.

With as little as five minutes, you can incorporate breathing exercises into your daily schedule in the morning, at lunch, or before going to sleep. The best part is that you can perform these techniques anywhere and anytime—a self-care tool for any occasion.

JOURNALING: A PATHWAY TO SELF-REFLECTION AND MENTAL CLARITY

Journaling is an important form of self-care that allows for self-analysis, self-reflection, and mental self-examination. Journaling allows us to describe our thoughts, feelings, and experiences in words; as we do this, we interpret how we feel and recognize patterns in our actions and reactions. This can be therapeutic in that it offers a space in which to release concerns, celebrate successes, and vent about our inner life without judgment.

Journaling comes in a number of shapes and sizes, each of which is beneficial. Gratitude journaling, for instance, can help take the edge off negative thoughts and improve mood by noting down what you're thankful for every day. Expressive writing—sharing openly your innermost thoughts and emotions—has been shown to reduce stress, improve mood, and even increase immune-system activity. Another popular option is the bullet journal, a user-configurable tool that merges to-do lists, goals, and journaling into an organized but fun exercise.

Journaling can be done once a day or on an as-needed basis. You need only a notebook (or an app on your phone) and a few quiet minutes, which should be accessible to anyone interested in taking better care of their minds. Journaling is a secure, private method of self-reflection, anger management, or simply chronicling the day.

MINDFULNESS APPS: DIGITAL TOOLS FOR ENHANCING SELF-CARE

Mindfulness apps are a great way to start incorporating self-care into your daily life. These apps feature guided meditations, breathing exercises, and other tools to cultivate mindfulness—the ability to stay alert and attentive in the present moment. A smartphone tap offers instant access to a wide array of routines that focus attention, lower stress levels, and enhance general well-being.

Popular mindfulness apps, such as IntelliCareAI, offer tools tailored to specific goals—reducing anxiety, encouraging sleep, or sharpening focus. These apps are generally full of tracking tools, reminders, and community forums to maintain motivation during the mindfulness exercise. The apps can be particularly helpful for introducing beginners to the concepts of meditation and breathing exercises and make these practices more approachable.

In addition to the primary benefits of mindfulness apps, a main draw is their convenience; they can be used from home, while on the road, or during a lunch break. This accessibility enables people to practice mindfulness during busy periods of the day. It can help users develop a more rounded mindset by investing even a few minutes of mindfulness each day, making life less stressful and them more resilient.

ADDRESSING NEGATIVE ONLINE INTERACTIONS: PROTECTING MENTAL WELL-BEING IN THE DIGITAL AGE

Negative online interactions like cyberbullying, trolling and abusive posts are very detrimental to mental health. With the online world immersing itself in our everyday lives, self-care is also about knowing how to control and guard against destructive online activity. This interaction can be full of anxiety and stress, and a source of feelings of failure, so you need to learn how to manage it effectively.

Having boundaries is one of the best ways to handle negative interactions online. These can be formed by restricting access to certain platforms, muting or blocking bad influencers, and filtering social media feeds for helpful content. Connecting with like-minded groups or interacting with well-being-minded accounts can create a better, more positive internet experience.

We also need digital detoxes—frequent disconnects from screens in order to reset the mind and break the dependency on perpetual access. In the case of an unpleasant interaction, disconnecting from the screen helps bring a sense of balance, and it averts automatic emotional responses. Another useful tool is positive affirmation and mindfulness techniques, like breathing or small-button meditation, to offset the adverse effects of negativity online.

Lastly, ask for help if you can, whether that be from friends, family, or licensed counselors who can offer support and guidance to handle all of these things. Putting mental health first and proactively monitoring online activities can help you have a healthier and happier online life.

The importance of self-care for mental, emotional, and physical health in a digital age is growing. Breathing exercises, journaling, mindfulness apps, etc. are quick and easy ways to reduce stress and increase mindfulness in your daily life. Fixing negative internet interactions and alternating screen time with movement and face-to-face socializing are also essential elements of a healthy self-care regimen. Combining these can lead to a better connection with technology, less exposure to digital stressors, and a more healthy, satisfying life. Not only does self-care boost well-being, but it also allows people to take on the challenges of modern life more tenaciously and cheerfully.

KEEPING SCREEN TIME IN CHECK WITH MOVEMENT AND CONNECTIONS

We live in a digitally consumed and physically demanding world, so the balance between the two is key to our sense of well-being. Excessive screen time—whether from social media, gaming, or office work—can create both physical health problems, such as eye strain, bad posture, and insomnia, and mental health concerns, such as anxiety and social isolation.

Exercise and face-to-face social interaction are important parts of self-care that can reverse these trends. Physical exercise is a great way to relieve the physical and mental stress caused by extended screen time. So too are social interactions in the form of actual physical human encounters.

Everyday activity—a walk at the edge of the park, an exercise class, or just some minutes of stretching—improves mood, enhances focus, and reduces stress. Moving away from the screen and opting for activities like outdoor sports, yoga, or dancing is not only good for your body, but it is also good for your mind. Taking frequent breaks, for example, to stand, stretch, or just walk around, can make all the difference to both your physical and mental performance.

Personal connection, belonging, and emotional support can all be enhanced through the human, face-to-face interaction that doesn't occur via digital communication. Socializing (for example, getting together with friends for coffee, going to a group exercise class, and participating in community activities) can enhance your life and sense of well-being.

MINDFUL AFFIRMATIONS

Mindful affirmations—positive thinking and self-empowerment—are intended to get your mind on a positive trajectory, inward-facing, and upholding self-knowledge and self-compassion. Infusing mindfulness principles, such as nonjudgmental awareness of present moments, with the power of uplifting words to yourself, can promote peace of mind, decrease stress levels, and improve mental health. Practicing these affirmations during your day can greatly influence your attitude and way of living.

There are many positive mental and emotional benefits of conscious affirmations. They help to nurture a positive, conscious state of mind by offering intentionally supportive words. Such utterances can be used to reframe negative thoughts, decrease stress, and increase self-compassion, all of which leads to a more balanced and durable lifestyle. By simply repeating affirmations voluntarily, participants can place themselves in the present and become calm and focused, overcoming anxieties and negative thoughts. This exercise makes people love and respect themselves, and it helps them get past their self-sabotage by strengthening their resolve and confidence. Affirming thoughts also facilitate emotional regulation, guiding individuals to act thoughtfully instead of impulsively when faced with difficulty.

Affirmations have the ability to change your thoughts long term, which helps you to think more positively and be more connected to yourself. Mindful affirmations are a simple but effective way to rewire our minds, hearts, and bodies and move us toward a peaceful and fulfilling existence.

In order to use mindful affirmations, start by choosing statements that are in accordance with your current needs and goals (for example, "I am calm and centered"). Sit quietly, breathe, and repeat the affirmations over and over, slowly and thoughtfully, focusing on the words and your feelings. Think about the good things and the feelings they evoke—peace or confidence. You can recite affirmations at any time during your daily waking time, such as while you're on your way to work or just before bed. Set reminders to do them—sticky notes or phone reminders. Ask yourself regularly how they make you feel; then adjust accordingly and pair them with meditation or journaling for an enhanced effect.

Consistency and patience are essential. Over time, these positive affirmations will help you to change your mindset, reduce stress, and maintain a positive outlook. Use apps like Mindful Affirmations to help. These tools provide options to focus your affirmations on a particular aspect of your life (family, relationships, etc.) at any given point in your life.

SUMMARY AND TO-DO LIST

To create a balanced schedule that's fit for all kinds of activities, find ways to limit screen time. This might include using apps that track and regulate screen time or defining times and places that devices aren't allowed, such as at meals or during the hour before bed. When we control our screen time and work on making sure there's more physical and social time throughout the day, we can truly lead a healthier and richer life. This can be accomplished through exercising, socializing, engaging in hobbies, or simply being outside in nature.

Smart Tips

Self-Care Checklist

1. **BREATHE MINDFULLY** (5-10 MINUTES)

2. **JOURNAL YOU THOUGHTS** (5-10 MINUTES)

3. **ENGAGE IN PHYSICAL ACTIVITY** (30 MINUTES)

4. **LIMIT SCREEN TIME**

5. **CONNECT SOCIALLY**

CHAPTER X

FINDING AND BUILDING SUPPORT NETWORKS

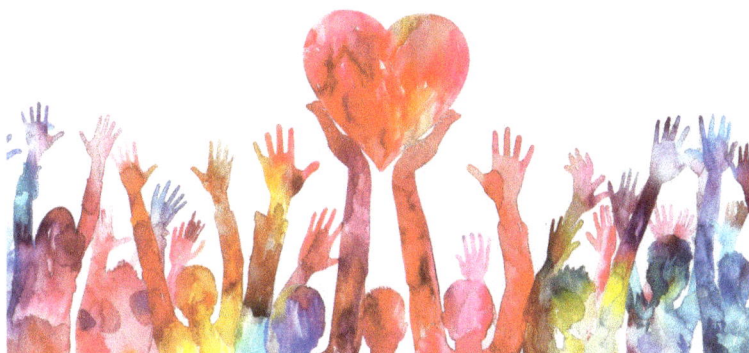

For teens, a strong support network isn't just nice to have—it's essential. Whether online or in person, being surrounded by those who uplift them can make all the difference.

—Lili Reinhart, Actress and Mental Health Advocate

Michelle Obama, in 2020, started a web project to support young people on social media and to help them locate positive networks that better their mental health. During her Becoming: Michelle Obama In Conversation series, she talked about the struggles of young people, especially during the pandemic, and how teens should have strong support groups. Michelle talked about how she thought social media could be embraced; she recommended adolescents "hang out with other people who share the same values, follow accounts that propagate good stuff, and get into groups that encourage conversation." She talked about having online communication with friends and family, particularly during stressful, lonely moments. Michelle focused on positive engagement and helped teens find social media networks that supported them, rather than tore them down, proving that social media approached with care can be an incredible resilience and mental health booster.

During a series of interviews promoted in October 2021, Twitter's cofounder Jack Dorsey affirmed his vision of how social media can be harnessed to form networks of support, particularly for mental health. He told one interviewer that "on Twitter, in particular, we've seen countless examples of how people—especially young people—can find a community made up of people who share their experience." He singled out two hashtags that have become a "call to action" around youth mental health—#MentalHealthAwareness and #YouAreNotAlone. These hashtags are used by tweens and teens to boost each other in the face of the shared challenges they face, giving voice to otherwise minor and silenced pains. "It began to invite teens into communities where they could find others around shared experiences of mental health," he said with a light touch of approval. He also invoked another Twitter initiative from 2018. If you type #MentalHealth in a tweet, Twitter provides a list of mental health resources. If you tweet a repetitive and unwanted pattern of negative thoughts, Twitter will invite you to find support and help.

Jack celebrated the positive ebb and flow of the force the social web can unleash as it fosters support circles amongst its users, even as it risks nudging them into adversarial relationships. The fundamental spearheading idea of Jack's message was that tweens and teens could be invited into communities where their truths would be heard and amplified—proving that, at minimum, a normative online ecosystem can indeed raise resilient, mentally healthy, caring, and connected youths.

S upport networks are crucial in helping teens navigate social media challenges and safeguard their mental health. These networks can provide guidance, encouragement, and a sense of belonging, counteracting the negative effects that digital environments can have on well-being. Effective support networks for teens must be built to help them manage social media use and protect their mental health.

INVOLVING FAMILY AS THE FIRST LINE OF SUPPORT

Family plays a fundamental role in a teen's support system, offering emotional security and guidance on healthy social media use.

Maintain Open Communication

Action: Encourage open, honest conversations about social media experiences. Create a safe space where teens can share their challenges, fears, and questions without fear of judgment or overreaction.

Purpose: Regular discussions help parents understand what their teens are going through online so that they can provide appropriate advice or intervention.

Set Boundaries Together

Action: Collaborate with teens to set realistic screen-time limits, establish tech-free zones, and discuss the importance of balancing online and offline activities.

Purpose: Working together fosters a sense of ownership and responsibility, making teens more likely to follow agreed-upon boundaries.

Model Healthy Digital Habits

Action: Parents should demonstrate mindful social media use, such as avoiding excessive screen time and not engaging in negative online behavior.

Purpose: Teens often mimic adult behavior; seeing parents set a good example helps reinforce positive habits.

LEVERAGING SCHOOL RESOURCES AND PEER SUPPORT

Schools are critical in supporting teens by providing education, resources, and peer-support programs.

Counseling Services and Support Groups

Action: Encourage teens to utilize school counseling services to discuss any social-media-related stress, bullying, or mental health concerns. Schools can also offer peer-support groups led by trained professionals.

Purpose: Professional support within the school setting provides teens with a trusted, accessible resource for managing social media's impact.

Digital-Literacy and Mental Health Education

Action: Schools should integrate digital-literacy and mental health education into the curriculum, teaching students about online safety, emotion regulation, and the signs of digital distress.

Purpose: Equipping teens with these skills empowers them to make informed decisions about their social media use and to seek help when needed.

Peer-Mentorship Programs

Action: Establish peer-mentorship programs in which older students guide younger peers on safe, healthy social media practices and provide a relatable support system.

Purpose: Teens often feel more comfortable discussing challenges with peers who understand their experiences, which fosters a supportive school culture.

BUILDING ONLINE SUPPORT COMMUNITIES

Online communities can provide a sense of connection and support, particularly for teens who may struggle to find understanding in their immediate surroundings.

Safe Online Spaces

Action: Encourage teens to join moderated forums, apps, or social media groups focused on mental health, wellness, or shared interests. Examples include platforms, like Discord, dedicated to mental health or specific subreddits offering peer support.

Purpose: These spaces offer a sense of community, reduce feelings of isolation, and allow teens to share experiences and coping strategies with others facing similar challenges.

Mental Health Apps and Resources

Action: Introduce teens to mental health apps—like Headspace, Calm, or Woebot—that provide resources, mindfulness practices, and even AI-driven mental health support.

Purpose: These tools help teens manage stress, anxiety, and social media's impact on their mental health in an accessible, on-demand format.

ENGAGING IN EXTRACURRICULAR ACTIVITIES AND COMMUNITY PROGRAMS

Involvement in activities outside of social media provides teens with valuable support networks and helps them build self-esteem and social skills in real-world settings.

Clubs, Sports, and Volunteer Opportunities

Action: Encourage participation in school clubs, sports teams, or community volunteer programs. These activities offer positive social interactions and reduce reliance on digital validation.

Purpose: Being part of a team or group fosters a sense of belonging, teaches teamwork, and provides a positive outlet for self-expression and connection.

Youth Groups and Community Centers

Action: Engage teens in youth groups, church activities, or community-center programs that focus on personal development, peer support, and leadership skills.

Purpose: These environments provide structured support and mentorship, helping teens build resilience and healthy relationships outside of the digital sphere.

CONNECTING WITH MENTAL HEALTH PROFESSIONALS

Professional mental health support is vital for teens struggling with social media's impact on their well-being.

Therapy and Counseling Services

Action: Encourage teens to connect with therapists or counselors who specialize in adolescent mental health and digital well-being. Many professionals offer virtual sessions, making it easier for teens to access support.

Purpose: Professional guidance provides tailored strategies for managing anxiety, depression, or other issues exacerbated by social media and offers a safe space to discuss and process emotions.

Support Hotlines and Online Therapy Platforms

Action: Introduce teens to resources—like Crisis Text Line, Teen Line, or online therapy platforms like BetterHelp and Talkspace—that offer confidential support tailored to young people.

Purpose: These services provide immediate help during times of distress and offer a convenient way for teens to access professional support without the barriers of in-person appointments.

EDUCATION ABOUT SAFE ONLINE INTERACTIONS

Building digital resilience involves teaching teens how to navigate online spaces safely and constructively.

Recognizing Red Flags

Action: Educate teens on identifying harmful interactions, such as cyberbullying, scams, or unhealthy comparisons. Provide strategies for blocking, reporting, and disengaging from negative encounters.

Purpose: Understanding how to handle harmful online behavior empowers teens to protect themselves and maintain control over their digital experiences.

Encouraging Positive Digital Citizenship

Action: Teach teens the importance of empathy, kindness, and respect in online interactions. Promote the idea of being a positive role model in their digital communities.

Purpose: Fostering positive digital citizenship helps create safer online environments and reinforces the importance of supportive, constructive behavior.

PARENT INVOLVEMENT IN BUILDING SUPPORT NETWORKS

Parents can actively help teens build and maintain support networks by connecting them with resources and encouraging healthy relationships.

Identify Trusted Adults and Mentors

Action: Help teens identify trusted adults, such as teachers, coaches, or family friends, who can offer additional support and guidance.

Purpose: Expanding a teen's network of trusted adults provides them with multiple sources of advice and reassurance beyond their immediate family.

Co-Navigate Social Media

Action: Spend time exploring social media platforms with teens, understanding their digital world, and offering guidance on how to handle challenges.

Purpose: Co-navigating social media helps build trust, provides an opportunity to teach safe practices, and reinforces the message that teens are not alone in their digital journey.

IMPORTANCE OF FINDING HELP WHEN NEEDED

Early Intervention
and Prevention

Counseling at an early stage can keep mental health problems from spiraling out of control. The sooner intervention is sought, the better the symptoms can be managed.

> **Impact:** Managing mental health issues early prevents long-term illnesses, enhances quality of life, and promotes improved long-term health.

How to Talk about Mental Health

- ✓ Choose right Time and Place
- ✓ Start with Empathy and Openness
- ✓ Be Direct but Gentle
- ✓ Normalize the Conversation
- ✓ Listen Actively and Without Interrupting
- ✓ Offer Support, Not Solutions
- ✓ Encourage Self-Care and Healthy Habits
- ✓ Follow Up

Professional Guidance and Expertise

Therapists, counselors, and psychologists offer expert advice, evidence-based techniques, and personalized treatment plans.

Impact: Professional assistance helps hone the skills to address a specific issue, develop strength, and change thought processes.

Validation of Feelings and Experiences

Reaching out for help provides validation that feelings and struggles are real and important. This validation is crucial for individuals who may feel misunderstood or alone in their experiences.

Impact: Having someone you can talk to who understands you helps lessen shame and stigma, promote open communication, and adopt a positive attitude about asking for help.

Coping Skills and Resilience Building

Mental healthcare providers facilitate the learning of coping skills that will manage stress, anxiety, and other mental and emotional conditions. Developing such skills provides resilience for future challenges.

Impact: Coping techniques promote emotional regulation and problem-solving, thereby mitigating the effects of future stresses on the brain.

Crisis Intervention and Safety

In times of crisis, such as severe depression, suicidal thoughts, or overwhelming anxiety, finding help can provide immediate intervention and safety measures.

Impact: Crisis support—such as hotlines, emergency counseling, or inpatient care—offers critical assistance when individuals are at their most vulnerable, preventing harm and providing a path to recovery.

Breaking the Cycle of Isolation

Seeking support interrupts the spiral of isolation that often looms over mental illness. Socializing with others who care about you and want to help eases loneliness and hopelessness.

> **Impact:** Building connections through seeking help reinforces the idea that no one has to face challenges alone and promotes a more connected and hopeful mindset.

SUMMARY AND TO-DO LIST

Developing support networks for adolescents is a key part of helping teens navigate the waters of social media and its potential effects on mental health. Through family, school, online groups, activities, and mental health professionals, teens can gain a complex support system to meet the specific demands and struggles they encounter. These groups can provide counseling, mentoring, and education services aimed at developing resilience, learning to cope well with

Smart Tips

Building Support Networks

1. UTILIZE ONLINE MENTAL HEALTH COMMUNITIES

2. SEEK OUT PEER SUPPORT PROGRAMS

3. EXPLORE THERAPY OR SUPPORT GROUPS

4. JOIN LOCAL CLUBS, CLASSES, OR MEETUPS

5. OPEN COMMUNICATION WITH TRUSTED ADULTS

stress, and forming a positive relationship with online resources. By creating healthy and positive spaces in these networks, teens become better equipped to make educated, healthier choices both on- and offline.

CHAPTER XI
SOCIAL MEDIA MONITORING

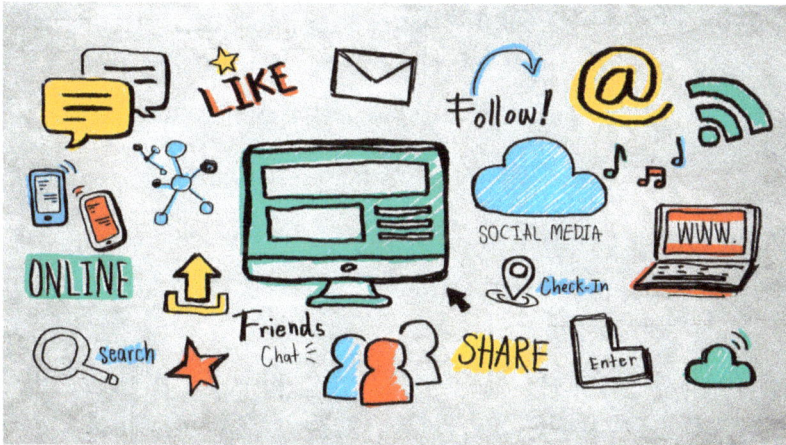

In an era of digital connectivity, monitoring social media is crucial for identifying potential threats and protecting public safety. However, it's equally important that we don't undermine trust and personal freedom in the process.

—Satya Nadella, 2022 CEO of Microsoft

Susan Wojcicki, former chief executive officer of You-Tube, described how she managed her kids' social media, emphasizing the importance of monitoring and guidance, "For me, being someone who's been a tech leader...helped me think about my kids' presence online. When kids started to use YouTube, they were excited by the opportunity and wanted to do it all day. So we monitored what kinds of videos they were watching... set rules around screen time...often watched them together and commented." It's possible that Wojcicki found it easier to undertake the parental-monitoring approach than others because she's the head of a platform that's been at the center of controversies around childhood well-being online.

But for most of us, monitoring kids' social media tends to be a strategy reserved for a specific set of situations. Because we have little time to spare watching what our kids post, we often approach monitoring with hesitant generosity so that it is not seen as an ultimatum fed to teens by helicopter parents.

Monitoring refers to tracking, analyzing, and sometimes intervening in individuals' online activities on platforms like Facebook, Instagram, Twitter (X), TikTok, and others to ensure safety, protect reputations, and manage risks associated with digital behavior. While this practice can offer significant benefits, it is important to note that, done incorrectly or too aggressively, it can present psychological, ethical, and practical challenges of its own, which can erode mental health, privacy, and trust.

HOW SOCIAL MEDIA MONITORING WORKS

Social media monitoring involves several tools and techniques to manage internet activity. This can be anything from simple checks to more complex programs that look for key words, hashtags, images, and geolocations in order to identify problematic behavior.

Parents keep track of their children's internet usage to safeguard them from cyberbullying, inappropriate online content, and predators. This might be via monitoring apps that offer reports on social media usage or parental blocks that lock out certain sites.

Employers monitor their workers to protect the company's image by tracing employees' online activity or that of job candidates to ensure they conform to company principles.

Schools keep tabs on students' activity on school computers or online in order to detect bullying, threats, or other signs of trouble.

Law enforcement agencies and governments search social media for threats, hate speech, crimes, or general public opinions.

POSITIVE IMPACT OF SOCIAL MEDIA MONITORING ON MENTAL HEALTH

Enhances Safety and Protection: Social media monitoring is a protective barrier for vulnerable populations like teens. By monitoring their online activities, parents and guardians can detect early signs of cyberbullying, self-harm, or predatory behavior. Early detection allows for timely intervention, potentially preventing long-term psychological harm.

Leads to Early Intervention and Crisis Prevention: Monitoring can serve as an early-warning system, alerting parents, schools, or mental health professionals to posts or behaviors that indicate a crisis, such as suicide ideation or extreme distress. In some cases, platforms have systems to detect harmful content and direct users to crisis helplines or mental health resources.

Encourages Digital Responsibility: Having the knowledge that your social media accounts are being watched can inspire more careful and responsible online behavior. This is especially relevant for younger users who might be unsure of the long-term implications of what they do online. Monitoring also encourages safety and responsibility.

NEGATIVE IMPACT OF SOCIAL MEDIA MONITORING ON MENTAL HEALTH

Privacy Invasion and Erosion of Trust: Constant monitoring can create a sense of surveillance that feels intrusive and violates personal privacy. This can damage trust between parents and children or employers and employees, creating an environment of suspicion. Individuals may feel as if they are always being watched, which can lead to anxiety, resentment, and even rebellious behavior.

Increased Anxiety and Self-Censorship: When someone knows their behavior is under surveillance, they might become suspicious of what they put online, how they interact, and even what they look up. This can lead to self-censorship and people not sharing what they really think or not interacting in a genuine way. Pressures to produce a "perfect" online image can lead to anxiety and negatively affect mental health.

Pressure to Conform and Fear of Judgment: Monitoring can exert pressures to meet certain requirements—particularly if you believe that you will be caught and penalized for any violations. Teenagers, particularly, may be compelled to repress their identity or passions in order to avoid conflict with adults, and this can be detrimental to their development and expression.

Dependence on Surveillance: More reliance on monitoring tools can shift the focus from fostering direct communication and digital literacy to simply watching and reacting. This reactive approach may miss opportunities to build trust, educate users about responsible social media use, and address the root causes of risky behavior.

Negative Effects on Self-Esteem: For those who are monitored, knowing that every action is under scrutiny can lead to decreased self-esteem. Constant correction or feedback, especially if not handled with care, can make individuals feel inadequate, incompetent, or unable to make sound decisions on their own.

BALANCING THE BENEFITS AND DRAWBACKS OF MONITORING

Achieving a balance between the benefits and psychological impacts of social media monitoring requires thoughtful implementation and a focus on mutual respect and understanding.

Open Dialogue: Honest conversations about the reasons behind monitoring and setting clear boundaries can help reduce the feeling of being surveilled. For parents and teens, discussing the risks of social media and agreeing on what is appropriate to monitor fosters a cooperative relationship rather than an adversarial one.

Use Monitoring as a Support Tool, Not a Control Mechanism: The primary goal of monitoring should be to support and protect, not to control. If concerning behavior is detected, approach it as an opportunity to provide guidance, education, and support, rather than solely focusing on punishment.

Empower Through Education: Be sure to not just focus on surveillance. Educate about digital safety, privacy, and what online behaviors affect. When people learn what social media is and how it can be dangerous, they can better utilize it responsibly.

Selective Monitoring: Consider targeted monitoring rather than blanket surveillance. For instance, monitoring only specific key words that relate to harmful behavior, rather than every single post or interaction, can reduce feelings of being constantly surveilled while still protecting against significant risks.

Respect Autonomy: You have to strike a fine line, especially between monitoring and respect for independence, especially with older teens and adults. Help those being monitored understand how important it is to be in charge of their digital lives, monitor themselves, and establish boundaries.

Social media monitoring, or the following and surveillance of social media networks for security threats, helps protect people and groups. It allows early intervention in cases of crisis, such as discovering and managing cyberbullying, self-injury, or harming other people. But we need to do this monitoring in a respectful and responsible manner, so as to prevent adverse effects on mental health.

A responsible social media monitoring strategy will include open communication, mutual respect, education, and encouragement. Open communication involves openly sharing the aim and methods of surveillance to build trust and transparency within the community being monitored. Respect is about taking into account the privacy and dignity of others, while observing and intervening only as necessary and appropriate.

SUMMARY AND TO-DO LIST

Social media monitoring is not meant to be intrusive or punitive. It should be an educational and supportive tool that helps the user understand what is in their social media histories and digital footprint. This understanding is the basis of any corrective measures needed to ensure that both their social media and digital footprint is a true reflection of themselves. Word clouds and risk profiles in the monitoring help in easily identifying how the world sees you and then taking appropriate corrective measures (if required).

Smart Tips

Social Media Monitoring

1. **MONITOR YOUR DIGITAL FOOTPRINT**

2. **SET CLEAR BOUNDARIES AND GUIDELINES**

3. **USE AS A SUPPORT TOOL, NOT PUNISHMENT**

4. **EMPOWER USERS WITH DIGITAL LITERACY**

5. **USE ALERTS AND MONITORING TOOLS**

CHAPTER XII

FUTURE-PROOFING YOUR DIGITAL LIFE

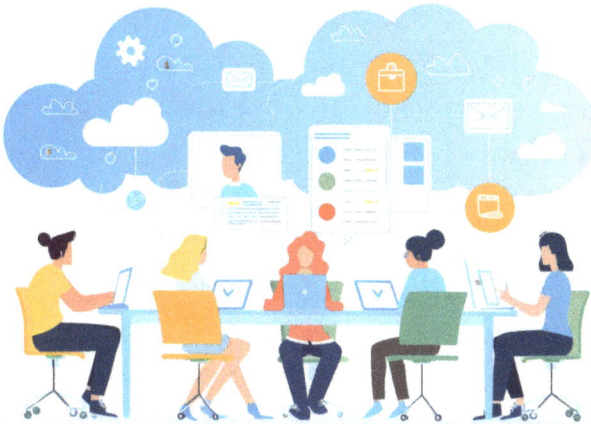

Future-proofing your digital life means embracing change and staying ahead of evolving technologies—adapting is the key to navigating an ever-connected world.

—Reid Hoffman, Cofounder of LinkedIn

In 2022, Satya Nadella, chief executive officer of Micro-soft, said to parents, "Make your teen future-proof," and he went on to say, "My wife and I are constantly thinking, 'How do we future-proof the digital life of our kids?' It's not just about, you know, let's monitor you, your hours logged into steam [a gaming platform], or whatever. It's about, 'Let's really invest in digital literacy and healthy tech habits. Let's think about pri-vacy settings; let's think about thinking before you hit Send; let's think about what you put on the internet will be used in your favor at some point in the future. It's a double-edged sword." Nadella is citing a stark reality in which human life in the information age constitutes a kind of precious heritage or legacy, and one's digital history can indeed "often be the most impactful sense of a person's history," as he says. So, for Nadella, we must teach our teens to manage their digital presences responsibly because in the informa-tion age, "that history will, at some point, open doors for you or close them." Here we have a high-ranking executive at one of the world's biggest technology companies explaining the necessity of "tell[ing] my kids what the right kind of digital footprint can do for them." Why doesn't Nadella see this advice as another aspect of what he calls "growing up digital in the future of work"—that is, another aspect of growing up under technocratic opioidism?

In 2021, Tim Cook, the CEO of Apple, spoke about the need to prepare teenagers for the reality of "future-casting" their digital lives. Speaking about some of the company's recent products, such as enhanced privacy settings and the Screen Time app, Cook emphasized how critical it is that today's teenagers have the knowledge and insight to "futurecast" their digital lives. In several televised interviews, Cook explained that Apple's vision is not to build products for parents that offer total control. Their goal, he explained, was to focus on offering products that encourage teenagers to take ownership of their digital footprint. Cook described the roles that his company's technical innovations play in teenagers' lives: they should be the digital "pyschos" who are helping young people to learn more about the data they are sharing and the potential opportunities or limitations it could create for their future "choice architecture." In essence, the concept of training teenagers as digitally literate citizens in the twenty-first-century public space is about equipping them with the knowledge and awareness to make informed decisions about their online actions so that they maximize their opportunities in the long run. Cook's focus was also on preparing them for the realities of their digital lives and drawing their attention to their level of futurecasting following their interactions on the various social media platforms available to them.

Digital future-proofing means securing your data, digital name, and online safety in the face of digital technologies and platforms. With our daily lives increasingly connected to digital content, you need to be resilient in the face of the next wave of cyberattacks and have a healthy online presence to further your personal and professional ambitions.

WAYS TO MANAGE YOUR DIGITAL FOOTPRINT

Your digital footprint contains all of the information about you that is on the internet. This includes your social media, posts, comments, photos and data you upload to sites. Being proactive with your online presence is vital because you have control over your online presence, and there is no possibility of giving away too much information.

Ask Yourself before Joining New Platforms
- ✓ What's the Purpose?
- ✓ What are my goals?
- ✓ Are My Privacy Settings Correct?
- ✓ Whom will I Interact with?
- ✓ What Concept Will I See?
- ✓ How Much Time Will I Spend?
- ✓ How Will It Impact My Health?
- ✓ Can I Easily Leave?

Regularly Audit Your Online Presence: You should always search for your name, email

168

address, and other personal data to make sure that it's not publicly accessible.

Google Alerts: Sign up for updates on any mentions of your name. Once you discover inaccuracies or sensitive data, you can ask that they be deleted. Then change your privacy settings, or do other things to protect your profile.

Minimize Personal-Information Sharing: Please do not post sensitive information on social media, forums, or online platforms. For privacy reasons, don't add details such as your house number, phone number, school name, or location. With a limit on how much data is published online, you will avoid identity theft, doxing, and other cyber harassment.

Clean Up Old Accounts and Content: Don't forget to go through and revoke or deactivate old accounts that you don't use anymore, like old social media accounts or blog pages. Delete or archive any old posts that are no longer yours or could be misinterpreted. When you streamline your online life, you reduce the chances of old or revealing content being republished.

Strengthen Digital Security: Cybersecurity is one of the most important components of securing your digital life in the future. With new cyberattacks a constant problem, good security habits help you secure your data and digital identity.

Use Strong, Unique Passwords and Password Managers: Use secure, unique passwords on each of your accounts. Don't use easily recognizable names or dates. Create and store complex passwords with a password manager. This will keep your accounts secure, particularly in case of data breaches compromising passwords.

Enable Two-Factor Authentication (2FA): Remember to enable two-factor authentication (2FA) for every account that supports it. This will provide a little more security because you will need to verify the identity with an additional method, such as a code you receive on your phone when logging in. This way, hackers are much less likely to break into your accounts, even if they can guess your password.

Monitor Accounts for Unusual Activity: Check your account activity for suspicious log-ins or changes. Configure notification alerts for new-account creation or other important account events. With alerts for unauthorized use, you can start taking measures right away to protect your accounts.

Keep Software and Devices Updated: Make sure your devices, apps, and software are up-to-date with all of the security patches and updates. Old software contains vulnerabilities that are easy for hackers to exploit, so upgrading your software often keeps you safe from new and emerging threats.

Curate Your Online Reputation: Your online reputation will affect everyone's opinion of you, be it when applying for jobs, college, or establishing your professional brand.

Build a Positive Personal Brand: Post content according to your values, interests, and work. Include projects, achievements, volunteer efforts, or other work that illustrates your abilities and personality. Creating an effective personal brand will make you stand out in the crowd and seem as if you are a trustworthy person within your niche or community.

Be Cautious of Controversial or Negative Posts: Do not post or engage in anything that is likely to offend, harm, or challenge. Before posting anything, think carefully about what employers, teachers, or other important people will see. You have to consider the potential long-term implications of what you do online and how you wish to project that image on the internet.

Utilize Privacy Settings: Don't forget to check and update the privacy settings on your social media accounts. This will allow you to control who can see your posts, photos, and information. Set them as Friends Only versus Public, if appropriate. If you control who can see your content, you will be able to preserve your data and stop others from stealing your information.

Be Skeptical of Sharing Sensitive Information: With data breaches, phishing scams and cybercrimes are escalating. It is important to think carefully about where and how you disclose sensitive data in order to secure your digital life in the future.

Limit Sharing of Personal Identifiable Information (PII): Please be cautious of submitting personally identifiable information (PII) such as Social Security numbers, banking information, or medical information. Only share this data when absolutely necessary, and then only through secure means. Providing personal data should be avoided in order to prevent identity theft and financial exploitation.

Beware of Phishing Scams: Avoid opening unsolicited emails, messages, or links that ask for personal information. Before clicking links or downloading attachments, confirm the sender's authenticity. Scams are becoming more sophisticated, and keeping up-to-date will protect your accounts and data from being hacked.

FUTURE-PROOF YOUR PROFESSIONAL PRESENCE

Future-proofing involves continually updating and curating your web presence. With changing professions and working landscapes, a professional online presence can help you thrive in the future.

Create a Professional Profile on LinkedIn: A clean LinkedIn profile increases your professional visibility, links you to job opportunities, and serves as a virtual resume.

Own Your Domain Name and Create a Personal Website: Remember to also register your name as a domain and have a personal website with your portfolio, projects, and career interests. If you own your domain, you can own the first page of search results for your name and make sure your professional narrative is being conveyed.

Maintain a Professional Image across Platforms: Make sure that you are posting in a professional way on your social media profiles, particularly those that potential employers or clients may see. Don't use unprofessional profile photos, and be careful about the tone and message of your posts. Having a consistent professional look and feel across platforms helps solidify your identity and lets employers or coworkers know that you're a good choice.

STAY INFORMED ABOUT
DIGITAL TRENDS AND RISKS

Cyberspace is never static, and new technologies, platforms, and threats are popping up all the time. Information allows you to adapt and protect your digital existence against emerging risks.

Follow Cybersecurity News: Check the cybersecurity news, blogs, and newsletters on a regular basis to keep up-to-date with the latest threats, such as scams, data breaches, and security vulnerabilities. If you are aware of these threats, you can take timely measures to secure yourself, such as changing passwords and adopting additional security protocols.

Understand the Privacy Policies of Platforms You Use: Check the privacy statements of your social media platforms, apps, and websites. You can then see what is being collected and stored with your data. Knowing what happens to your data will allow you to make educated decisions regarding which platforms you work with and how you manage your data.

Learn About Digital Detox and Mental Health: Take the time to learn new habits like digital detox, which is disconnecting from your screen and recharging your body and mind. Know the effects of digital overstimulation on your psychological well-being. By separating your digital and offline life, you avoid burnout and stress, and improve overall well-being, so that your digital life doesn't physically, mentally, and emotionally drain you.

SUMMARY AND TO-DO LIST

Ensuring the longevity and security of your digital presence demands continuous attention and effort. This involves vigilance in monitoring and refining your online footprint, employing robust security protocols, taking deliberate steps to shape and maintain your online image, and staying updated on the latest developments in the digital sphere. By consistently managing these aspects, you can effectively adapt to the dynamic digital environment while fortifying your online persona and protecting your personal and professional interests.

Smart Tips

Future-Proofing Your Digital Life

1. **KEEP YOUR DEVICES AND APPS UPDATED**

2. **USE STRONG PASSWORDS AND 2FA**

3. **ORGANIZE AND BACK UP YOUR DATA**

4. **BE MINDFUL OF WHAT YOU SHARE ONLINE**

5. **STAY INFORMED ABOUT DIGITAL TRENDS**

— CHAPTER XIII —

YOUR PATH FORWARD

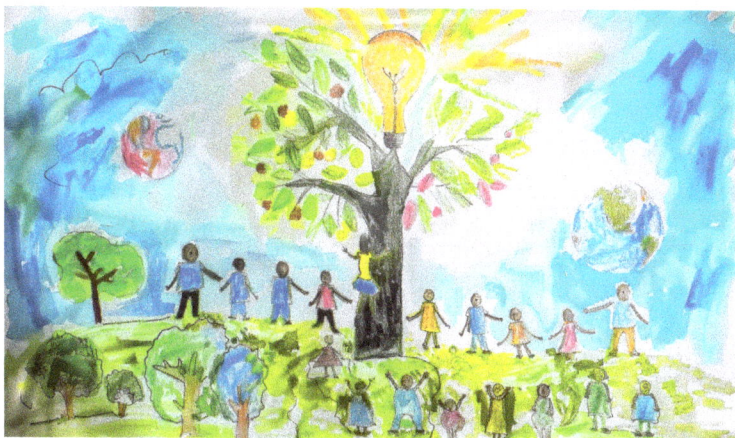

As we navigate our digital future, prioritizing safety and well-being will ensure technology remains a tool for connection, not a source of harm.

—Prince William, Duke of Cambridge and Mental Health Advocate

Adolescents can be very excited but terrified when it comes to social media. Social media provides teens with a different kind of space in which to interact, learn, and communicate. But the virtual world can also be a risk to their mental and emotional health. The teenager has to find a middle ground between making the most of social media and being mindful of their mental health in order to protect their well-being in this digital age. So they must use a few strategies to get on the right side of social media while still protecting their mental health.

First and foremost, they must adopt a healthy and mindful mindset with their online behavior. That means being aware of how social media can affect their mood and self-confidence. Also, teens must focus on quality over quantity in the online relationships they engage with—meaningful and supportive connections, rather than validation in the form of how many followers or likes they have.

In addition, teens can help set tech-free time periods in their schedule to turn off social media and do other activities (for example, exercising, reading, or hanging out with friends and family). By setting limits on how socially connected they want to be, teenagers will have a more balanced relationship with social media.

PRACTICE MINDFUL SOCIAL MEDIA USE

Set Intentions: Encourage teens to use social media with purpose—connecting with friends, exploring interests, or learning something new. Avoid mindless scrolling that can lead to wasted time and negative emotions.

Limit Screen Time: Set healthy boundaries around social media use, such as taking regular breaks, avoiding use during meals, study times, and before bedtime to reduce overuse and prevent sleep disruption.

CURATE A POSITIVE AND AUTHENTIC ONLINE EXPERIENCE

Follow Positive Influences: Encourage teens to follow accounts that inspire, educate, or bring joy and to unfollow or mute those that cause stress, comparison, or negativity.

Be Authentic: Promote sharing real moments, not just the highlights. Authentic self-expression can reduce the pressure to maintain a perfect persona and foster genuine connections.

BUILD AND ENGAGE IN SUPPORTIVE COMMUNITIES

Connect with Trusted Friends and Family: Strengthen connections with people who provide support and encouragement, both online and offline. Engaging with a trusted network reduces reliance on social validation from strangers.

Seek Safe Online Spaces: Encourage participation in moderated groups or communities that are focused on shared interests or support and where interactions are respectful and uplifting.

DEVELOP CRITICAL THINKING AND DIGITAL-LITERACY SKILLS

Distinguish Reality versus Highlight Reel: Teach teens to recognize that social media often showcases the best moments of others' lives, not the full picture. Encourage them to avoid unhealthy comparisons and remember that everyone faces challenges not shown online.

Question Content and Intent: Educate teens on how algorithms work and why content is shown to them. Critical thinking helps them discern between genuine, helpful content and manipulative, misleading posts.

RECOGNIZE AND MANAGE NEGATIVE EMOTIONS

Identify Emotional Triggers: Encourage teens to reflect on how social media makes them feel. If certain interactions, accounts, or content consistently cause distress, they should adjust their use or take a break.

Use Social Media Tools: Platforms offer features like muting, blocking, and limiting screen time. Teach teens to use these tools to protect their mental health and control their digital environment.

PRIORITIZE OFFLINE ACTIVITIES AND REAL-WORLD CONNECTIONS

Balance Digital and Real Life: Encourage teens to engage in offline activities—such as sports, hobbies, volunteering, and spending time with friends and family—to build confidence and resilience outside the digital world.

Foster Face-to-Face Interactions: Real-world connections provide authentic support and validation, helping teens feel valued beyond their online presence.

SEEK HELP WHEN NEEDED

Talk About Challenges: Encourage open conversations about the connections between social media experiences and their mental health. If social media negatively impacts their well-being, remind teens that it's okay to seek help from trusted adults, counselors, or mental health professionals.

Utilize Mental Health Resources: Direct teens to apps, hotlines, and online resources that offer support, coping strategies, and professional guidance tailored to young people.

CONCLUSION

To sum up, by being mindful of social media and adopting good strategies, like screen-time limits and breaks, adolescents can make use of the positive features of social media while also protecting their mental well-being. In this healthy manner, they can enter the online world confidently, securely, and with health in mind, aware of what they're doing and how it might affect their mood and self-confidence.

The way forward for teens on social media is a balance between the positive by being part of a community and using positive content, the negative by not sharing personal information and limiting screen time, and the mental by seeking support and taking time out when feeling overwhelmed. By using social media mindfully, curating content that offers value, following stories that are useful and motivating, and reaching out when needed—either to parents or professionals—teens can use social media to bring meaning to their lives while still protecting their mental health.

Smart Tips

Your Path Forward to a Digital Future

1. BE SELECTIVE ABOUT WHAT YOU SHARE

2. ENGAGE POSITIVELY AND MINDFULLY

3. KEEP YOUR PROFILES UPDATED

4. MONITOR YOUR DIGITAL FOOTPRINT

5. SECURE YOUR ACCOUNTS

CHAPTER XIV

HELPLINES, APPS, AND OTHER RESOURCES

Helplines and mental health apps remind us that support is always within reach, even in the darkest moments. They are essential tools for healing and connection.

—Michelle Obama, Former First Lady
and Advocate for Youth Mental Health

WHAT ARE HELPLINES?

Helplines, also known as hotlines or crisis lines, provide immediate crisis counseling, emotional support, and information at no cost. Most helplines have toll-free numbers, and many also offer support through text messages or online chats. They are often available twenty-four seven, so you can access help whenever you need it, day or night.

Mental Health Hotlines

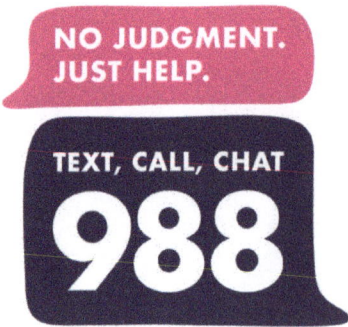

National Suicide Prevention Lifeline (US)

Phone: 988

Website: 988lifeline.org

Free 24/7, confidential support for people in distress, harm-prevention and crisis-counseling resources.

Crisis Text Line (US, Canada, UK, and Ireland)

Text: HELLO to 741741

Website: crisistextline.org

Free 24/7 text support from trained crisis counselors.

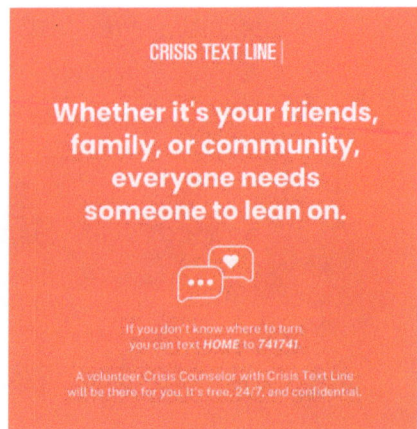

SAMHSA National Helpline (US)

Phone: 1-800-662-HELP (4357)

Website: samhsa.gov

Free confidential information and treatment referrals for mental health and substance-use issues.

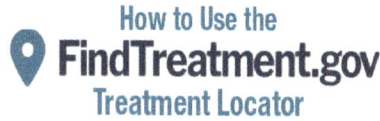

How to Use the

◉ FindTreatment.gov

Treatment Locator

Need to find treatment for mental and substance use disorder in your area?
Go to **www.findtreatment.gov** and follow these easy steps:

◉ FindTreatment.gov

Lifeline (Australia)

Phone: 13 11 14

Website: lifeline.org.au

Free 24/7 crisis support and suicide-prevention services.

MENTAL HEALTH APPS

Mindful Affirmations

Platform: Web, iOS (coming), Android (coming)

Guided meditations and mindfulness affirmations to produce a positive mindset.

Headspace

Platform: iOS, Android

Mindfulness and positive-affirmation tools for mental health and wellness.

Calm

Platform: iOS, Android

Meditation, breathing exercises, sleep stories, and music for relaxation.

BetterHelp

Platform: iOS, Android, Web

Connects users with licensed therapists for online therapy sessions via chats, videos, or phone calls.

Talkspace

Platform: iOS, Android, Web

Online therapy with licensed professionals through live sessions, messaging, or both.

Woebot

Platform: iOS, Android

Mental health chatbot that provides emotional support and cognitive behavioral therapy (CBT) techniques.

MENTAL HEALTH WEBSITES

NAMI (National Alliance on Mental Illness)

Website: nami.org

Mental health resources, support groups, and educational materials.

Mind (UK)

Website: mind.org.uk

Information on mental health issues, support options, and ways to seek help.

Mental Health America

Website: mhanational.org

Mental health screening tools, resources, and information on finding support.

7 Cups

Website: 7cups.com

Free emotional support through anonymous chats with trained listeners and licensed therapists.

ReachOut (Australia)

Website: reachout.com

Resources, tools, and support for teens and young adults facing mental health challenges.

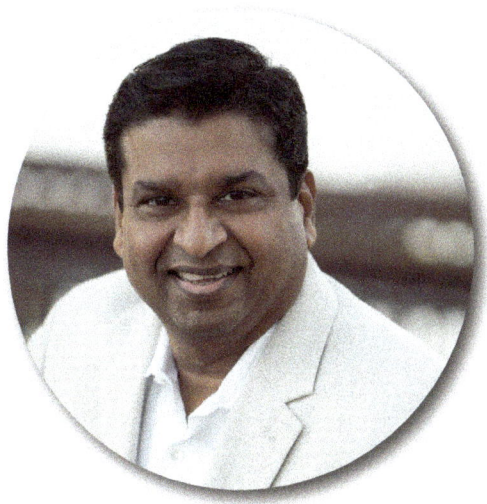

LET'S CONNECT

Hubert A. Jerome

www.hubertjerome.com

hjerome@hubertjerome.com

www.navigatingthedigitalmaze.com

www.facebook.com/navigatingthedigitalmaze

www.instagram.com/navigatingthedigitalmaze

MY SAFE SCHOOLS

A groundbreaking platform that is transforming student safety and wellness through five innovative modules:

Thrive delivers essential life lessons tailored for teens, enhancing their education and personal growth.

Safe Social monitors social media interactions to protect digital well-being and promote positive online behavior.

Speak Easy allows students to anonymously report concerns, fostering strong and supportive communities.

IntelliCare leverages cutting-edge AI tools to provide personalized wellness solutions, ensuring each student receives the care they need.

CALM offers in-house live counseling and life-management services, comprehensively addressing emotional and psychological well-being.

Together, these modules create a secure and nurturing environment where every student can thrive. My Safe Schools empowers the next generation to stay safe, healthy, and successful—making schools better for everyone.

www.mysafeschools.com

info@mysafeschools.com

https://www.instagram.com/mysafeschools

https://www.facebook.com/mysafeschools

https://twitter.com/my_safeschools

https://www.linkedin.com/company/mysafeschools

INTELLICARE AI

Where innovation meets wellness, IntelliCare AI is a cutting-edge app dedicated to enhancing your mental health and wellness journey. Powered by an advanced AI mental health platform, IntelliCare AI offers personalized support through mindful affirmations, guided meditation, and journaling tools. You can set and achieve your wellness goals with features designed to foster emotional resilience and balance. Whether you're looking for daily motivation, stress management, or simply a space in which to meditate, IntelliCare AI, your mental wellness partner, gives you the tools to flourish and live your healthiest, happier life.

www.interllicareai.com

info@intellicareai.com

https://www.instagram.com/intellicareai/

https://www.facebook.com/intellicareai

THRIVE PUBLICATIONS

Thrive Publications—Life Lessons for Teens

The *Thrive* series from My Safe Schools equips teens with practical insights and vital life skills, from managing relationships and emotions to cultivating healthy habits and making significant decisions.

www.thrivepublications.org

info@thrivepublications.com

www.instagram.com/thrivepublications

www.facebook.com/thrivepublications

MY WORD CLOUD

My Word Cloud—See How the World Sees You

In today's digital world, your online presence matters more than ever. Our cutting-edge technology and expert analysis delivers a clear picture of your social media footprint, ensuring that your online reputation aligns with your personal or professional goals.

www.mywordcloud.com

info@mywordcloud.com

www.instagram.com/mywordcloud

www.facebook.com/mywordcloud

www.ingramcontent.com/pod-product-compliance
Lightning Source LLC
Chambersburg PA
CBHW040254290326
41929CB00051B/3380